Advancing Responsible A

MW01092684

Editor:
Roger J.R. Levesque

Faye Z. Belgrave

African American Girls

Reframing Perceptions and Changing Experiences

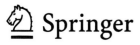 Springer

Prof. Faye Z. Belgrave
Virginia Commonwealth University
Department of Psychology
806 W. Franklin St.
Richmond VA 23284
Box 841218
USA
fzbelgra@vcu.edu

ISBN 978-1-4419-0089-0 (hardcover)   e-ISBN 978-1-4419-0090-6
ISBN 978-1-4614-1517-6 (softcover)
DOI 10.1007/978-1-4419-0090-6
Springer Dordrecht Heidelberg London New York

Library of Congress Control Number: 2009926173

Cover Design: Frido

Printed on acid-free paper

Springer is part of Springer Science+Business Media (www.springer.com)

Preface

Over the past 15 years, I have had the opportunity to conduct research and intervention programming with African American girls. Several of my graduate students, mostly African American women, pursuing their doctorates in psychology worked closely with me in this work. We have conducted hundreds of literature reviews, read many journal articles and reports, published many papers, and engaged over a thousand African American adolescent girls in a cultural curriculum specifically designed for them. This book was written to summarize this work and was conceived to be an educational resource for diverse audiences who work with African American girls including: (1) researchers who conduct research and intervention programming; (2) professionals who work with African American adolescent girls such as teachers, social workers, prevention specialists, therapists and counselors, and mental health workers; and (3) a general audience of persons with an interest in African American adolescent female's well-being and development such as parents, community leaders, girl's group leaders (i.e., Girl Scout leaders), and church and spiritual leaders.

This book is both descriptive and practical. Each chapter covers the most current literature on African American adolescent girls, and reviews and discusses ways in which they are similar to and unique from girls in other ethnic groups and from African American boys. An understanding of who they are and how they function allows us to make recommendations about ways to support these girls and to refocus and/or strengthen already positive attributes. A related purpose is to begin to address some of the disparities African American girls face (i.e., teen pregnancy, HIV infection, obesity, etc.).

There are three parts to this book. The first part, "Who Am I" provides an introduction to the remainder of the text (Chap. 1) and how African American females view themselves (Chap. 2). The second part on "How Did I Come to Be" includes both proximal and distal influences on African American girls' behavior and well-being. This part discusses her family and kin (Chap. 3), friends and peers (Chap. 4), and community (Chap. 5). Community peers and families have a great influence on her expectations and achievement, and a chapter on achievement and expectations is also included in this part (Chap. 6). The third part 'Who Will I Become' discusses contemporary issues facing African American girls that impact her health, social, and overall well-being. Chapters on health and wellness (Chap. 7), sexuality

(Chap. 8), and pro-social behavior and aggression (Chap. 9) are addressed in this part. Chapter 9 is followed by concluding comments.

My hope is that the reader will be inspired to attend to African American girls with a sharper focus on her strengths, her talents, and other assets.

Richmond, VA   Faye Z. Belgrave

Contents

Part I

Chapter 1
Description and Demographics

Over the past 15 years, I have had the privilege of working with thousands of African American adolescent girls who have participated in our prevention interventions and who have been involved as participants in research studies we have conducted. Additionally, colleagues and I have had both formal and informal discussions and interviews with many African American girls. Sometimes, I have simply observed them in their daily activities while they were in school, attending after school programming, and in community and religious activities. My learning has also come from personal interactions and experiences. I have 1 daughter, 12 nieces, and 2 goddaughters whose lives I have been a part of. This book is about these girls, who they are, their achievements, their dreams, their hopes, and to some degree their failures.

I wrote this book with two goals in mind. The first goal is to highlight the resiliency and strengths found among African American adolescent girls. Although there is variability, African American girls generally possess high self-worth, confidence, and assertiveness. They assume responsibilities within their families and are guided by spiritual and religious beliefs and behaviors. African American girls engage in prosocial behaviors, including kindness and charity to others. They hold high expectations regarding academic achievement and most believe they can do well.

At the same time there are many problems our girls face. While their academic achievement is higher than that of African American males, it is lower than that of girls from most other ethnic groups. Early and unprotected sexual activity among many of our girls results in teen pregnancy, parenting, and sexually transmitted infections. Additionally, there have been recent increases in use of certain drugs and in aggressive acts. Childhood obesity and other poor health outcomes are also of concern as these health outcomes establish a trajectory for poor health as adults. Therefore, my second goal of writing this book is to present the research and data regarding these problem areas to bring attention to them.

This book presents the most recent research and literature on African American girls. It is about: (1) how we can refocus and strengthen the energizing force in our girls; (2) how positive behaviors can be encouraged and negative behaviors can be eliminated by drawing upon inner strengths and natural ways of being; (3) how we can work collectively through families, schools, communities, and other institutions to support positive development of our girls; and (4) what girls can do themselves

F.Z. Belgrave, *African American Girls*, Advancing Responsible Adolescent Development, DOI 10.1007/978-1-4419-0090-6_1, © Springer Science+Business Media, LLC 2009 to strengthen their spirit and well-being. To accomplish these goals, a recommendation and resource section is included at the end of each chapter. This section provides examples of exercises and activities that can be used across diverse settings to promote well-being and positive functioning.

Universal and Divergent Perspectives

African American girls are both similar to and unique from other groups. There are traits, values, and behaviors that African American girls share with all girls and with African American boys. For example, she is relational as are most females. She is also likely to have a communal worldview which is found among most persons of African descent. A relational and communal worldview assumes that others are important to her sense of self and general well-being, and that her attitudes and behaviors are influenced by others. Her gender role beliefs tend to differ from those of girls in other ethnic groups in that she possesses both instrumental (e.g., masculine) and expressive/nurturing (feminine) gender role beliefs. These androgynous gender role beliefs may be shared by African American boys. While she shares many values and behaviors with African American boys, there are also differences. For example, her academic achievement and life-course expectations tend to be higher, and she is more likely to finish high school and graduate from college. These and other universal and divergent perspectives will be presented and discussed throughout this book.

African American girls' socioenvironmental context also influences who she is and who she will become. Her family, the closest and most immediate influence, has a profound impact on her current and future actions. Many African American girls grow up in low-resource urban communities, and these settings may contribute to lower expectations and achievement and sometimes deleterious outcomes, such as early parenting. Gender, race, and class discrimination also exist within this country and have adverse effects on her well-being.

Who this Book is About

This book focuses on African American adolescent girls primarily those in early and middle adolescence between the ages of 10 and 14. During this period, there are many biological, social, and psychological transitions. Puberty begins during this period; there is transition from elementary to middle school; and girls began to develop friendships and interests outside the home. Interests in romantic relationships begin as does sexual identity. During this developmental period, girls have an increased desire for independence in decision making as they begin to think abstractly and reason logically. This can be an exciting time in her life and also a period of problems and turbulence. Whether or not her transition is successful has long-term consequences for her life-course trajectory. Decisions made during this vulnerable period can have both positive and negative consequences for the rest of her life. For example, girls who do well academically during this period are likely to continue to do well in high school and beyond. Those who begin to struggle academically may establish a cycle of failures that erodes academic persistence. Girls who become teen parents face many challenges, economically, socially, and personally later in life. Research and literature on her well-being, behaviors, and functioning across several domains are examined along with literature on factors that promote and attenuate behaviors and well-being.

Heterogeneity Among African American Girls

African American girls are not all the same and to represent them that way would be to stereotype. Like all Americans, they live in rural, suburban, and urban communities; are members of families of varying socioeconomic levels; and engage in different levels and types of prosocial and problem behaviors. In reviewing literature and research, the majority has been written and published on urban girls, probably because the majority of African Americans live in urban areas. Research and literature on girls from diverse environments and circumstances is presented in this book to the extent possible. Each chapter summarizes and discusses current research and literature on African American adolescent girls highlighting issues that are most salient and relevant to their well-being and ways of functioning. Many of the chapters reference work I have done with graduate students and colleagues. A discussion of African American girls begins with a discussion of African Americans in the United States.

African Americans and Blacks in the United States

Where African American girls live and the socioeconomic conditions of their families (i.e., income education, poverty, etc.) are sociocultural factors that contribute to their well-being. An overview of some relevant demographics among African Americans in the United States is provided next.

According to the United States Census, Black or African American refers to "A person having origins in any of the Black racial groups of Africa." It includes people who indicate their race as "Black, African American, or Negro" or provide written entries, such as African American, Afro American, Kenyan, Nigerian, or Haitian. In this book, the term "African American" is generally used. In some cases, the term "Black" is used to retain the intent of the author cited.

African Americans comprise 12.8% of the United States population. When Black is considered with another racial or ethnic group, African Americans comprise 13.4% of the US population. According to the United States Census (2007), in 2006 there were approximately 40,000,000 persons who were Black/African American singularly and/or in combination with other racial/ethnic groups. This represents a percentage increase of 8.5% since 2000 (U.S. Census Bureau, 2007).

Where do African Americans Live?

In 2004, almost 60% of African Americans lived in ten states: New York, Florida, Georgia, Texas, California, Illinois, North Carolina, Maryland, Louisiana, and Virginia. African Americans are more likely to live in the South than in any other region of the country. Approximately, fifty-four percent lives in the South, 19% in the Midwest, 18% in the Northeast, and 10% in the West. Geographically, African Americans are concentrated in urban areas or cities. The ten cities with populations greater than 100,000 with the highest percentages of Blacks are: Gary, Indiana; Detroit, Michigan; Birmingham, Alabama; Jackson, Mississippi; New Orleans, Louisiana; Baltimore, Maryland; Atlanta, Georgia; Memphis, Tennessee; Washington, D.C.; and Richmond, Virginia.

Family Structure

African American girls live in extended and intergenerational families that often include grandparents. According to the U.S. Census Bureau, 35.2% of African American girls live in married-couple households, 54.4% live in mother-headed households with no husband present, 7.5% live in mate-headed households with no wife present, and 2.9% live in nonfamily households (U.S. Census Bureau, 2007 American Community Survey Reports). About 20% live in households with grandparents.

Socioeconomic Indicators

About 80% of African Americans aged 25 and older are high school graduates, and about 17% have a bachelor's degree or a higher level of education (U.S. Census Bureau, 2004). In terms of occupations, about 27% of African Americans are employed in management/professional occupations or in sales and office occupations. About 23.5% of African Americans are in service occupations. The remainder is employed in occupations, such as construction, transportation, and farming. About 54% of African Americans own the homes they live in compared to the total population percentage of about 76%.

The April 2009 unemployment rate for African Americans over the age of 20 was 15% compared to a rate of 8% for Whites and 3.2 for Asians (U.S. Bureau of Labor Statistics, 2009). The ethnic differential in the rate of unemployment is substantial for individuals between 16 and 19 years of age with an unemployment rate of 34.7 for African Americans and 19.7 for Whites. About 24.9% of African Americans live poverty compared to the national percentage of 12.5. In African American female-headed households, close to 27% live below the poverty line (Devanas-WaH Proctor, & Smith, 2008).

African American Children and Teens

In 2006, there were approximately 3,246,000 African American teens between the ages of 10 and 14 and 3,359,000 teens between the ages of 15 and 19 (U.S. Census, 2007). These numbers represent 16% of all US teens in the 10 to 14-year-old age group. Similarly, African American teens between the ages of 15 and 19 represent 16% of all teens in this age range. African American children are overrepresented among those who live in poverty. Close to 35% of African American children live in poverty. These statistics show that about 1 out of three African American girls live in poverty.

Overview of Chapters

This book is organized in three parts. The first part "Who am I" is an introduction to the book and how African American females view themselves. The second part "How did I come to be" covers both proximal and distal influences on African American girls' behavior and well-being. This part covers her family, her friends and peers, and her community. Her community, peers and families have a great influence on her expectations and achievement, and a chapter on achievement and expectations is also included in this part. The third part "Who will I become" covers contemporary issues facing African American girls that impact her health, social, and overall well-being. Chapters on health and wellness, sexuality, and prosocial behavior and aggression are addressed in this section.

Part 1: Who am I?

African American girls' view of the self and her identity are discussed in Chapter 2. Several aspects of her identity are covered, including self-worth, self-complexity, ethnic or racial identity along with relational values, gender roles, and sexual identity. Research suggests that African American girls have fairly high feelings of self-worth and confidence, and androgynous gender roles that comprise both high masculine and feminine beliefs. Along with androgynous gender role beliefs, cultural attributes such as ethnic identity protect girls, especially those who may encounter stressors due to community disadvantage.

Part 2: How did I Come to Be?

Chapter 3 covers several topics relevant to African American families, including who is in her family, what her family looks like, her roles within the family, family discipline, communication and conflict with mother and father, monitoring, and racial socialization among other topics. African American girls live in diverse and extended families that often include grandparents. She is likely to have positive and fulfilling relationships with her mother and father, and these protect her from some of the adverse challenges that arise from institutional and neighborhood obstacles.

The influence of friends and peers is discussed in Chapter 4. Friends are important to the psychological and social well-being of all adolescent girls. Friendship patterns among African American girls are similar to those of girls from other ethnic groups with some exceptions. Overall, adolescent girls have more friends than boys. While there is sometimes mistrust of other girls, African American girls tend to maintain intimate friendships. Like girls from other ethnic groups she tends to select friends who are similar with some exception. Romantic relationships also begin to occur during the period of early adolescence. The chapter also touches upon the topic of interracial friendships.

Communities and neighborhoods are more distal than the family but very influential to African American girls' well-being. Communities and neighborhoods are discussed in Chapter 5. Many African American girls live in low-resource communities. Neighborhood disorganization, poverty, and socioeconomic disadvantage have pervasive and negative effects with regard to stress levels, health, and drug use. Communities also affect academic achievement and expectations although less for African American girls than boys. Youth who reside in urban versus rural communities face some similar and unique challenges, and these are too discussed. Schools and teachers as community institutions also impact African American girl's academic achievement and other outcomes. Included in Chapter 5 is a discussion of factors that attenuate the effect of community disadvantage on girls.

Research has shown that the type of community that a girl lives in affects her future expectations and achievement, and this is the topic of Chapter 6. African American females tend to have higher academic achievement and expectations when compared to African American males; reasons for this are also discussed in this chapter. Her expectations for education, getting married, and having a baby are different from those of girls from other ethnic groups as her expectation for age for having a baby is lower and her expectation for age of marriage is higher. Her expectations are influenced to a great degree by parents, especially the mother's expectations and communication with her daughter.

Part 3: Who will I Become?

This first chapter in this part of the book, Chapter 7, addresses health and wellness among African American girls. This chapter provides an overview of health issues among African American teens. It begins with a discussion of puberty which brings on many biological, social, personal, and psychological changes. African American girls tend to enter puberty at a younger age than girls from other ethnic groups, and one sign of this is an earlier age of menstruation. African American girls have poorer dietary and fitness habits than girls in other ethnic groups. Poor diet and fitness activities are contributors to elevated rates of obesity and diabetes among African Americans. Also, African Americans have high prevalence and morbidity from asthma, and this is discussed. Regarding mental health, African Americans are similar to girls from other ethnic groups and show increases in depression levels from early to late adolescence. Drug use is also discussed, although being an African American girl is actually a protective factor against drug use. However, when African American youth do use drugs the consequences of drug use are much worse. Girls tend to use drugs because of relational reasons of wanting to belong, fit in, and be accepted by others. Culturally integrated drug prevention programs have been successful in decreasing drug use and increasing drug refusal efficacy among African American girls.

Sexual behaviors and consequences are discussed in Chapter 8. Outcomes from early and risky sexual behavior are of concern. African American adolescent females engage in higher levels of sexual activity than most other ethnic groups and initiate sex at an earlier age. Outcomes from unprotected sex include early parenting with concomitant social and economic stressors along with increased risk for sexually transmitted infections and HIV. African American girls tend to use condoms more than girls from other racial and ethnic groups but remain at higher risk because of the level of HIV infection in the African American community. There are several risk and protective factors associated with early and risky sexual activity, and they are reviewed in this chapter. The chapter also provides suggestions for preventing early and risky sexual behavior.

Chapter 9 discusses the topics of prosocial or helpful behavior and aggression. This chapter reviews literature on determinates of prosocial behavior, including empathy and perspective taking. These factors are similar for African American girls and girls from other ethnic groups. However, cultural factors, such as communalism, and religion and spirituality also contribute to prosocial behavior. Chapter 9 also covers aggression and violence by and against girls. African American girls are more likely to be the victim of partner violence rape and date rape, and believed to be less credible when this violence is reported. Concluding comments by the author are presented following Chapter 9.

Recommendations and resources are provided at the end of each chapter. The recommendation and resource section is especially designed for those who work with African American girls, including educators, social service workers, recreational workers, and parents. Many of the suggested activities can be implemented in a variety of settings, such as schools, community agencies, recreational facilities, churches, and homes. The recommendations and resource section might also be of value to researchers and program implementers who are looking for effective strategies and programs. Recommendations are in the form of suggested activities and exercises, and discussion topics. The nature and type of information varies. In some cases, recommendations are informal ones that are readily available on the internet. In other cases, evidence-based and empirically supported interventions are described along with contact information.

Chapter 2
Self and Identity

*I love it. I love it. Even if I knew before I was born and I had a
choice, to be any other color, black, Indian, anything, I love
being black. It's just something about that. I mean, even though
I know how my race is considered in the media and to other
eyes, to other races or whatever, I love my race. I mean I would
not change it for anything. I love everything about it. I love my
skin color. I love black people, I mean they [White people] got a
different way of doing things.*[1]

13-year-old African American girl

The above quote is from a girl who was asked what she likes about being African
American. Although she is aware of the negative media portrayal of her race, she
strongly identifies with being African American and has a strong emotional attachment to Black people. In this chapter, several aspects of the self, including racial
or ethnic identity, gender roles, relationships, and sexuality, are discussed. The
chapter examines how African American female adolescent's views of self impact
other important self attributes, including self-esteem, self-complexity, risky sexual
behavior, body image, and sexual identity.

One of the primary tasks of adolescence is to develop an identity. Our identity is
derived from our past experiences, defines who we are, and who we will become. A
central component of our identity is the feelings and beliefs we have about our self.
Ways of thinking about the self have been termed "self-concept," "self-liking," "self-
esteem," "self-complexity," and "self-worth." Other aspects of our identity include
how we feel about being male or female, and how we feel about the ethnic or racial
group to which we belong. Our sexuality is another aspect of our identity.

Our identity develops in response to what is going on in the immediate (family)
environment as well as the environment outside the home, including schools, communities, religious institutions, and the larger society. The media also has a powerful
influence on the development of our self and identity. The process by which identity develops is called "socialization." This process begins at birth although it is not

---

[1] Interviews were conducted by the author or colleagues with African American girls between the
ages of 11 and 16. These girls resided in two metropolitan areas on the East Coast.

F.Z. Belgrave, *African American Girls*, Advancing Responsible Adolescent Development,
DOI 10.1007/978-1-4419-0090-6_2, © Springer Science+Business Media, LLC 2009

until there is self-awareness that identity development can be tracked. For females, identity development also evolves through an understanding of the self in relation to others (Miller, 1991). For females, identity involves the roles and expectations of being a female. For African Americans, it also involves feelings, beliefs, and behaviors about being a person of African descent.

Self attributes, including self-esteem and self-worth, are discussed next, followed by a discussion of ethnic identity, relational orientation, gender roles, body image, sexuality, and a chapter summary. The "Recommendations and Resources" section of the chapter provides suggestions and activities that can be used to increase self-concept and other aspects of identity.

The Self

What is the Self and what does it Mean to Adolescent Girls?

By self, we mean the conscious awareness of one's own being or identity as an object that is distinct from others (Baumeister, 1999). Self-concept is our beliefs and thoughts about who we are. A teen with a positive self-concept believes that she can get along with others, that she can do well in school, and that she has special talents and abilities. Much has been written about the decline in positive self-concept among adolescent girls. One reason for this decline is that negative images and expectations from the external environment become self-confirming as girls began to internalize the beliefs that they feel others hold of her. While her perception of negative views from others may not be accurate, they nonetheless may become self-fulfilling and subsequently positive actions and achievements decline. The self-fulfilling cycle starts with a negative self-concept which promotes negative behavior and, in turn, reinforces a negative self-concept. The opposite occurs in the case of a positive self-concept. Positive actions and achievements set the stage for continued positive self-concept and achievements, which lead to even more positive accomplishments. As we will see, the development of the self differs for African American girls than girls from other ethnic groups, and her conceptualization of herself is generally positive.

Self-concept may be especially vulnerable during early adolescence between the ages of 11 and 14. There are several critical changes that occur during this period. School transition from elementary to middle or junior high school is a major event that occurs during this period. The less restrictive school environment along with additional responsibilities may not provide the structure to support girls in maintaining a positive self-concept. As will be discussed in subsequent chapters, other transitions that occur during early adolescence include puberty, and increased relationships and activities with peers. In overview, the many and varied social, biological, and relationship changes that occur during this period can negatively impact her self-concept and identity.

Self-Concept Among African American Girls

The beginning of adolescence may bring on a more negative self-concept for girls from most ethnic groups; however, research shows that this does not occur with adolescent African American girls, at least not to the same extent (Greene & Way, 2005). This is not to say that some African American teens do not have negative self-concepts, but overall their self-concepts tend to be positive. In our assessment of self-concept among thousands of African American teen girls, we have found self-concept to be positive across several domains such as appearance, getting along with others, doing well in school, and in physical and athletic achievements (Belgrave; Corneille & Belgrave, 2007).

Girls, who have participated in intervention programs and research studies we have implemented, tend to report high self-confidence (Belgrave et al., 2004; Corneille & Belgrave, 2007). In both interviews and paper-and-pencil surveys, African American girls have reported positive self-attributes such as confidence, high self-esteem, high self-worth, and confidence in their ability to problem solve and cope with adversity. Their beliefs about their abilities to do well across a variety of tasks are generally positive. Later in this chapter, I return to why this may occur sometimes in the face of adversity. We can build upon the tendency of African American girls to have positive self-concept and strengthen it even further.

What are Other Aspects of the Self?

Self-esteem is another aspect of the self. Self-esteem is liking (or disliking) of the self and involves a favorable (or unfavorable) assessment of the self in areas that are important. Self-esteem differs from self-concept in that self-concept encompasses beliefs and thoughts about the self, while self-esteem refers to feelings and affective evaluations about the self. Self-concept and self-esteem differ but are related. Low self-esteem brings about bad feelings, while low self-concept brings about bad thoughts. Self-esteem has to do with being satisfied with who you are and with feeling good about who you are. Self-esteem may include a girl's assessment of her appearance, school grades, ability to make friends, or other attributes important to her. Girls might like or feel good about how they look, how they get along with members of their family, and how well they do academically. We have found that African American girls tend to have high self-esteem along with high self-concept.

Do African American Girls Assume Multiple Roles?

Self-complexity is the extent to which one sees oneself as having several or few dimensions or aspects to one's life (Linville, 1985). For African American teen females, self-complexity could include different dimensions such as being a daughter, a student, a member of the band, or a good friend. Persons high in self-complexity see themselves along several dimensions, and persons low in self-complexity see themselves primarily along a few dimensions. For example, a girl with low complexity might see herself primarily as a student or a daughter.

African American adolescent girls are relatively high in self-complexity as they report on several dimensions of importance to them. They see themselves as a member of both their immediate and their extended family, as a member of their church or religious congregation, and as a member of their friendship group. They also see themselves as a student, and as a member of a number of other community and neighborhood groups. Overall, high self-complexity can be positive. If a person is failing in one domain of the self, then they are less likely to experience negative emotions if they do well in other domains that are important to them (Linville, 1985). For example, if a girl receives a failing grade in school (a domain that is important to her) but she sings a beautiful solo in the church choir (another domain important to her), she will be less devastated by the low grade than if she only saw herself as being a student. The negative side of high self-complexity occurs when the individual has competing demands, roles, and responsibilities on her time (i.e., being a good student, daughter, friend, and the responsibilities each of these positions require).

Why is Self-Concept and Other Aspects of the Self Generally Positive Among African American Girls?

Positive attributes of the self among African American females are likely due to her socialization within the family, extended family, and church or other religious institution. Many African American parents racially socialize their children (Stevenson, 1995). Racial socialization messages involve telling children how to function in the larger society and also how to function as an African American. Racial socialization messages for girls involve preparing them for womanhood. For example, parents may tell their girls to "get an education." African American mothers may also tell their daughter to "get an education so that you can take care of yourself and not be dependent on others." Thomas and King (2007) conducted a study that examined specific socialization messages given to African American daughters by their mothers. They found that mothers provide different types of messages to their daughters. These messages had themes of self-determination, pride, and religion.

Messages with spiritual and religious themes may stress the value and sacredness of all life regardless of job, education, or position in life. From an African-centered perspective, one's value and worth is not based on materialistic things and acquisition of positions or power but in service to God and family and community. The socialization of these values may be adaptive for African American girls. Her involvement in spiritual and religious activities also promotes and maintains her self-esteem and self-concept by providing institutional settings in which girls are connected to and supported by each other. Messages of pride and self-determination were instilled when parents spoke of how their forefathers and foremothers survived and thrived under oppressive circumstances and that they therefore should be able to survive in the face of adversity. These messages are also likely to promote high self-concept and ethnic identity.

Racial and Ethnic Identity

Ethnic identity is our connection to persons who are ethnically or racially similar to us and is linked to our self-concept. Although racial identity and ethnic identity have been used interchangeably, they differ. Racial identity is based on one's identification as a member of a racial group, and ethnic identity is based on one's identification as a member of an ethnic group. Race is based on biological perception and ethnicity is based on social and cultural perception. The term "ethnic identity" is used mostly in this book.

What is Ethnic Identity?

Ethnic identity is one's feelings toward and identification with an ethnic or racial group. For African Americans, the degree of ethnic identity is determined by whether the person feels attached to or connected to African Americans and other people of African descent (Phinney & Kohatsu, 1997). African Americans with strong ethnic identity feel good about being of African descent; they desire to be with other African Americans, and they engage in behaviors that support these feelings and desires. For example, African Americans with high ethnic identity prefer to shop in Black-owned stores and use Black-owned services. A person with a negative ethnic identity engages in practices that are associated with Whites as Whites are their primary reference group. They affiliate with Whites and believe Blacks are not as competent as Whites. They also might assume that poverty and poor conditions among African Americans are due to their own fault, perhaps believing that African Americans lack motivation or that they do not take advantage of opportunities (Helms, 1990).

Most African Americans function on a continuum of low-to-high ethnic identity. They may feel positive about being African American in some dimensions but not in others. For example, they may feel that it is ok to go to an African American physician for health care but feel that a predominately African American school is not as good as a predominately White school. We have observed that girls who have been in our intervention and research projects tend to have moderate levels of ethnic identity. One of the goals of our intervention programs has been to increase ethnic identity (Belgrave, Reed, & Plybon, 2004).

Why is Ethnic Identity Important for African American Girls?

Research has shown that high ethnic identity is associated with many positive behaviors and favorable outcomes among African American adolescent girls (Corneille & Belgrave, 2007; Marsiglia et al., 2001; Townsend & Belgrave, 2000). Girls with high (compared to low) ethnic identity use fewer drugs and have attitudes that are intolerant of drugs (Belgrave, Brome, & Hampton, 2000; Burlew, Neely, & Johnson, 2000). They are less likely than girls with low ethnic identity to become sexually active at a young age and are more likely to protect themselves from pregnancy and sexually transmitted infections (Belgrave et al.). The positive benefits of ethnic identity are also seen in better school performance and better social relations with friends. Finally, persons with high ethnic identity are more likely to engage in prosocial behavior and to be helpful to others (Smith, Walker, & Fields, 1999).

Low ethnic identity is associated with misconceptions of Africa and what it means to be of African descent. Girls with low ethnic identity may want to distance themselves from Africa and African Africans. They may assume a superior attitude regarding people and things that are African centered. When this occurs, efforts can be directed toward correcting these misperceptions. Strategies we have used are discussed in the "Recommendations and Resources" section. Relationships are important to the development of self and identity and are central to African American adolescents. Relationships are discussed next.

Relationships

An interpersonal relationship is a connection or bond between two or more persons. Relationships serve social and intimate needs as well as instrumental and task-oriented needs. Our first significant relationship is with our parents and then with others outside our family and kin. Relationships are especially important to the well-being (or lack of) of females.

Why are Relationships Important to African American Girls?

Most females, old or young, African American or Asian, rich or poor, are relational in orientation (Miller, 1991). This means that relationships are valued and needed for her well-being. Relationships can be with family, friends, teachers, other supportive adults, God or other spiritual or religious figures, and romantic partners.

A girl's relationship with others contributes to a large extent to the development of her identity during the period of early adolescence. While relationships are also important to boys, the way in which relationships influence identity differs for boys than girls (Miller, 1991). During the period of early adolescence, boys seek to establish autonomy and independence from others. Their sense of who they are is independent from others, while a girl's sense of self is interdependent on others. A girl's sense of self is determined by how others see her and what others expect from her. If significant others provide her with information that she is a person of value and worth, her beliefs about her self will be positive. If significant others provide her with information that she is not valued, then her beliefs about herself may be negative. The nature and quality of her relationships with significant others are important in her identity development. The person who is likely to be most influential in her development is her mother but could also be her father, grandparents, cousin, teacher, or other supportive adult.

Given the importance of relationships among girls, particularly during early adolescent development, significant others can be a source of positive or negative influence. If relational needs are not met in a mutually fulfilling positive relationship, then there may be attempts to get these needs met within destructive and negative relationships. Girls who do not have positive relationships with their parents and other family members are more likely to engage in risky and delinquent behaviors than girls who have positive relationships within her family. Girls with poor family relationships are more likely to fare poorly in school, engage in drug use, and engage in early and risky sexual activity (Miller, Forehand, & Kotchick, 1999; Travis & White, 2000).

What does a Relational Orientation Mean for African American Adolescent Girls?

Interdependent relationships are very important to girls. Relationships with adult females help to guide their sense of self and their behavior as these relationships provide them with models of what to expect and how to behave. Relationships are also important to people of African descent. A central worldview among most people of African descent is communalism which is akin to a relational orientation. Communalism from an African-centered perspective considers that African American family and community experiences are characterized by interpersonal relationships, group identity, and shared relationships (Hurley, Boykin, & Allen, 2005). Thus, while relationships are important to all females, they may be especially so to African American females given the relational values of both people of African descent and females. Another aspect of a girl's identity is that of herself as a female and what it means to be a female in this society. This has been referred to as "sex roles" or "gender roles" and is discussed next.

Gender Role Beliefs

An adolescent girl's thinking about what is and is not appropriate behavior for a girl/boy or man or women has implications for her choices and behaviors along many dimensions. How she acts within her family, her coursework and success at school, her activities within the community and church, and her career choices are all affected by her gender role beliefs.

What are Gender Role Beliefs?

Gender role beliefs are the expectations and beliefs that people hold as to how males and females are supposed to feel, think, and act (Bem, 1993). These beliefs can typically be categorized as "masculine" or "feminine." Sometimes, words such as "independent" and "instrumental," or "nurturing" and "expressive" are used to describe gender role beliefs associated with masculinity and femininity, respectively. When people are described as independent, assertive, willing to take risks, a leader, and decisive, they are said to have masculine or instrumental gender role beliefs. People described as emotional, attentive, caring, cooperative, and helpful, are said to have feminine gender role beliefs.

Gender Role Beliefs Influence Attitudes, Expectations, and Behaviors

Girls with instrumental gender role beliefs may engage in more risky and daring activities, and participate in activities that are traditionally associated with masculinity, such as taking engineering and math courses in school. Girls with feminine gender role beliefs are more likely to seek traditionally feminine careers such as teaching and nursing. They are also more likely to take care of others, show concern for the welfare of others, and be emotionally expressive. Girls with feminine gender role beliefs may not want to assume leadership positions and may not be drawn to traditionally male-oriented careers. Both masculine and feminine gender role beliefs can be positive, or these beliefs can inhibit or limit girls in certain activities. In general, females tend to have more expressive gender role beliefs and males more instrumental. However, as will be later discussed, this is not the case with African American girls.

It is possible to measure gender role beliefs with questions such as "Are you emotional?" "Are you caring?" and "Do you like being around children?" (Spence, Helmreich, & Stapp, 1974). Individuals who agree with these items are considered to have expressive or feminine gender role beliefs. Masculinity questions might include items such as "Do you like to take charge?" "Do you care about others' opinions?" and "Are you competitive?" It is possible to score high on both instrumental and expressive traits and behaviors. These individuals are considered androgynous. Individuals who score low on both masculine and feminine items are considered undifferentiated.

Children develop gender role beliefs through socialization where they learn from their parents, teachers, friends, the media, and the larger society about what it means to be a male or a female in this country. Gender role socialization starts at birth. For example, infant boys may be allowed to cry longer than infant girls in an attempt to toughen boys up. We can also observe gender role socialization in the types of toys that are provided for young children. Girls are given dolls to care for and boys are given trucks to explore the world with. When girls and boys act in gender-appropriate ways, they are often praised and rewarded.

Why are Gender Role Beliefs Important?

Gender role beliefs ultimately affect the choices we make and how we behave. Girls with feminine gender role beliefs may limit themselves in terms of the academic courses they take, the career they choose, and the decisions they make about relationships. In relationships, girls with feminine gender role beliefs may feel that it is the male's responsibility to make decisions about the relationship, including decisions about sexual activity. Girls with feminine gender role beliefs may also be more likely to seek out a vocation or career that is traditionally female. These might include careers in education, social service, or other helping positions. Girls with feminine gender role beliefs may be less likely to seek out careers and jobs in traditionally masculine occupations, such as engineering, construction, etc.

Researchers have speculated that instrumental gender role beliefs are beneficial for girls. For example, girls who are assertive may be likely to speak up in class and subsequently perform better. However, the beneficial effects of instrumental gender roles may depend on the context. In one study, we found that African American girls with higher instrumental gender role beliefs had riskier sexual attitudes than those with lower instrumental gender role beliefs (Belgrave et al., 2000). Perhaps girls with high (as compared to low) instrumental gender role beliefs are also more likely to engage in more rebellious and risky behavior, such as drug use and early sexual behavior.

What are the Gender Role Beliefs Among African American Adolescent Girls?

African American females, both adults and teens, tend to be androgynous more so than traditionally feminine or masculine (Ashcraft & Belgrave, 2004; Way, 1995). This means that they tend to have both high masculine and high feminine beliefs. This is not to say that all African American adolescent girls are androgynous, but they are more so when compared to girls from other ethnic groups. Research also suggests that African American boys may be more androgynous than boys from other ethnic groups (Harris, 1996).

There are several reasons why African American adolescent females tend to have androgynous gender role beliefs. A combination of masculine and feminine gender role beliefs has enabled African American females to succeed within the family and workforce despite a history of racism and discrimination. Historically, African American females have had to take responsibility for the well-being of herself and her family. She is typically employed, and is often the one who makes housing and other purchasing decisions singularly or in cooperation with her partner. These types of instrumental activities are carried out while she cares for her children, extended and elderly family members, and sometimes neighbors.

The lack of employment opportunities for African American males may also be a contributing factor to African American women developing androgynous gender roles, beliefs, and behaviors. Good employment opportunities are not as available for African American men as women and African American women are more likely than African American men to complete high school, and to attend and graduate from college (U.S. Census Bureau, 2007: American Community Survey Reports). Thus traditional gender role beliefs seen among men and women of other ethnic groups may occur less so among African Americans because gender differences in employment and education tend to favor African American women. In fact research suggests that gender role beliefs conform to beliefs about social roles (e.g., homemaker versus employed) that men and women hold (Eagly & Steffen, 2000).

Finally African American girls learn from and model androgyny from others. They are exposed to their mothers, grandmothers, and other female role models and adopt the beliefs and behaviors of these women. They see women who are simultaneously involved in caring for others, achieving economic and employment self-sufficiently, and in making independent decisions. They are often told to get an education in order to get a job to take care of yourself.

What does it Mean to be Androgynous?

A fair amount of research has been conducted on what it means to be androgynous (Ashcraft & Belgrave, 2004; Harris, 1996; Woodhill & Samuels, 2003). Studies have found that African American girls who are androgynous have higher levels of self-esteem and ethnic identity, and engage in less risky drug use and sexual risky behaviors compared to girls who are not androgynous. Androgynous girls (from all ethnic groups) tend to have better mental health and psychological functioning than girls who are feminine or masculine (Buckley & Carter, 2005; Rose & Montemayor, 1994). They have higher self-esteem, higher self-worth, and are more confident. These girls are also more likely to choose academic subjects and careers that are more challenging.

In general, girls who have participated in our intervention and research projects can be described as androgynous. They think, act, and display behaviors that are both "independent" and "nurturing." Another salient aspect of identity for adolescent girls is their body and the image they have of it. This is discussed next.

Body Image

Body image is an often-discussed topic as it relates to adolescent girls' self-esteem and other aspects of the self. Body image is both perceptions of body size and beliefs and feelings about physical attributes (Cash & Pruzinsky, 1990). According to a survey by Kid Source (1998), physical appearance is "extremely" or "very" important to most girls' self-esteem.

Why is Body Image Important?

A girl's perception of her body image is directly associated with positive and negative feelings about the self. These feelings and beliefs in turn influence behaviors. Girls with poor body image have lower self-esteem, lower feelings of self-worth, and are more likely to be depressed (Brausch & Muehlenkamp, 2007; Santos, Richards, & Bleckley, 2007). Negative body image perception is also linked to anorexia, bulimia, and other types of eating disorders. The link between negative body image perception and poor functioning is true for African American girls as for girls from other ethnic groups (Siegel, 2002; Wingood, Diclemente, & Harrington, 2002). Girls with a positive body image have positive feelings about themselves and are likely to spend time on self-improvement activities, thereby continuously increasing positive body image.

   In one study, researchers looked at how body image was related to risky or protective sexual behaviors among African American adolescent females (Wingood et al., 2002). The authors found that females who were less satisfied with their body image were more likely to fear abandonment when negotiating condom use and more likely to feel that they did not have as much control in their sexual relationships. In other words, negative body image may precipitate feelings about being a desirable (or undesirable) partner. Girls who do not feel that they are desirable dating or romantic partners may feel that they have less room to negotiate in the relationship.

Ethnic Differences in Body Size Perception

Historically, African American girls have been less concerned about their body image than White and Hispanic girls (Jones, Fries, & Danish, 2007). African American girls are less likely to diet and to engage in other weight management practices such as exercise and subsequently may have fewer eating disorders. However, this is changing and today we see more African American females with dissatisfaction about their bodies. Striegel-Moore (2003) found that young black women were as likely as white women to report binge eating. In an earlier study, Striegel-Moore (2000) found that black women were as likely as white women to report binge eating or vomiting and were more likely to report fasting and the abuse of laxatives or diuretics than their White peers. Thus, negative beliefs about body image may adversely affect African American girls more so than previously believed.

On the other hand, African American girls are more accepting of a larger body size for themselves and others (Jones & Crawford, 2005). A larger body size acceptance can be healthy and eliminate obsessive worry about being thin. However, larger body size acceptance can encourage obesity, a leading contributor to chronic health conditions such as diabetes among African American females.

African American Adolescent Females and Skin Color and Hair Texture

"If you are black, stay back, brown, you can stick around, and white, you are all right." This saying was frequently used during my childhood to distinguish who was and was not a person of worth based on skin color. In addition to body size and shape, skin color and hair are two physical attributes that impact African American girls and women. There is also a great range in African American people with regard to these two physical attributes. Although beliefs about skin color and hair texture are changing somewhat, historically, it has been considered desirable to be light skinned and to have straight hair (contrasted with kinky hair) (Hill, 1998; Hunter, 2002; See & Larkin, 2007). Studies have found that African American women who are lighter and have straighter hair are considered more attractive. And in the not too distant past, lighter skin females have been able to obtain higher levels of education and employment income than women who were dark skinned. When self-conceptualization is based on Eurocentric attributes (i.e., light skin, straight hair), girls who do not possess these attributes may have lowered self-worth, a contributing factor to risky and negative behaviors.

How does the Media Influence Self-Perception of African American Adolescent Females?

Although there are some exceptions, media targeting African American girls still use European standards of beauty where attractiveness is seen as thin bodies and long straight blonde hair. Hip-hop music targeted at teens may be especially influential in shaping body image and appearance perception. Girls with continual exposure to the models shown in music videos may contrast these models to themselves with resulting erosion of perceptions of self-beauty. Fortunately, there is some hip-hop music with positive messages.

Additionally, African American women may be stereotyped on television and portrayed as sex objects by the music industry. Messages from some rap songs and songs that are degrading to women contribute to a negative self-conceptualization

(Littlefield, 2008). Gordon (2004) found that media portrayal of African American women as sex objects was associated with African American adolescent girls' feeling worse about themselves and with self-concepts that focused on appearance and romantic ideas. Racial identity along with religiosity and parental involvement somewhat buffered girls from these beliefs. The media exposure to girls with high ethnic identity did not have the same effect of lowering their feelings of self-worth as it did for girls with low ethnic identity. A final aspect of identity to be discussed is sexual identity.

Sexual Identity

Sexual identity speaks to how one views the self as a sexual being, including sexual orientation (Diamond, 2002). During the period of preadolescence, sexual identity becomes salient. African American girls face the same problems of developing a sexual identity as girls from other ethnic groups with the added challenges of handling other identity issues. Her ethnicity, neighborhood, and contextual environment can potentially interfere with her progress toward accepting her sexual identity.

The development of an African American girl's sexual identity is based on the messages and meanings she is given about sexual roles and behaviors. Stephens and Phillips (2003) discuss how scripts unique to adolescent African American females' experiences have been framed within a racialized and sexualized sociohistorical context. They note that the historical Jezebel, Mammy, Matriarch, and Welfare Mother images of African American woman remain today, as exemplified by similar, yet more sexually explicit scripts that include the Diva, Gold Digger, Freak, and Dyke. The African American female Diva is one who has an attitude and who expects to be adored. Divas are high maintenance and spend a lot of time on appearance and looking good. A Gold digger is a woman who is materialistic and desires money above all else and is willing to trade sex for money. A Freak is a woman who is sexually aggressive; she desires sex without emotional intimacy. Women who reject sex from men are considered Dykes. This is based on the assumption that women are innately sexually oriented only to men.

Another aspect of sexual identity is sexual orientation. The percentage of all lesbian, gay, and bisexual (LGB) youth who self-identify during early adolescence is not known (D'Augelli, 2006). Early adolescents who are LGB have to function within the two primary social settings, the home and school. And they sometimes are confronted with stigma and hostility within these social settings. Sexual orientation and other identity issues can be especially challenging for teens, including African American girls.

Sexual minority individuals undergo the unique developmental process of coming out and developing a positive sexual identity as a lesbian or a bisexual woman. There has been limited work on coming out and developing a positive sexual identity as a lesbian or a bisexual female (Rostosky, Danner, & Riggle, 2007). However, some evidence from small samples of sexual minority adults suggests that an individual's religiosity may be a deterrent in the coming out process and the achievement of a positive sexual identity (Rostosky, Danner, & Riggle, 2007). Many religious institutions are intolerant of LGB individuals, and strong affiliation with these institutions may be a source of conflict. Therefore, for African American girls, who are lesbian or bisexual, higher levels of religiosity may interfere with positive sexual identity development and exacerbate health risk behavior rather than provide a protective effect or developmental asset. Many lesbian and bisexual girls run the risk of social stigma and isolation which affects the development of relationships important during early adolescence.

Life-Course Expectations

Our identity has a large effect on life-course expectations. Life-course expectations are the expectations that one has for what will happen in adult life. These include expectations about graduating from high school, attending college, when to become a mother, when to get married, and what kind of career or job one will hold. Life-course expectations and how these expectations affect academic, career, social, and family outcomes are discussed in more detail in Chap. 7.

Summary

African American girls' conceptualization of self and identity is complex and multi-dimensional. Self-concept and identity are important to consider as these beliefs affect who she is and who she will become. In many ways, development of the self and identity for African American girls follows the same trajectory as girls in other ethnic groups. In other ways, it differs.

In general, African American adolescent girls tend to have high self-concept, self-esteem, and self-complexity. She has moderate levels of ethnic identity, and ethnic identity may be negative if she has not learned to value being of African descent. African American girls value relationships, and their identity is closely linked to these relationships. Relationships can have both positive and negative influences. If relationship needs are not met in a positive mutually fulfilling relationship, they may be met by more destructive negative relationships. African American girls tend to be androgynous which means that they score high on both masculine and feminine beliefs and behaviors. Overall, androgynous gender role beliefs are adaptive as they are linked to several favorable outcomes. Recently, African American girls have reported poorer body image, in part due to negative media portrayals. Identity development among girls who are lesbian or bisexual is challenging and may present conflicts within the home, school, and religious institutions.

In conclusion, African American girls' have resiliency and strengths along several dimensions of the self. Her self-conceptualization is influenced by factors and circumstances that are both positive and negative. In the next section, suggestions for strengthening self attributes are provided.

Recommendations and Resources

The activities, exercises, and discussion topics that follow can be used to enhance an African American girl's sense of positive self and identity. We have used many of these activities with girls who have participated in our intervention programs. Some of the suggested activities are available off the internet and are in the public domain. Consistent with a relational orientation, most of these activities are best done within a group setting. These activities can be implemented by a parent, teacher, program facilitator, or supportive adult.

Increasing Positive Affirmations and Relationships

The objective of this activity is to increase a girl's positive regard for herself and others in her group. This exercise is best done with an on-going group of girls who know each other or who have met at least once or twice.

Provide each girl with a sheet of paper and have each girl write her name at the top. Then have every girl in the group write one positive word that comes to mind when thinking of each girl in the group. Encourage girls to think about behavior and attributes rather than physical appearance. For example, "she shares her lunch" or "she is generous" rather than "she has a great hair style." At the end of this exercise, each person has a list of positive affirmations that they can refer to from time to time. This exercise helps each girl learn how to say positive things about others and how to receive positive messages about themselves.

An alternative way of doing this exercise is to have girls gather in a circle. Each girl would say a positive word about the girl to her left (or right). This allows all the girls in the group to hear positive messages. This exercise also contributes to the development of group cohesion.

Promoting Ethnic Identity

The objective of these activities and exercises is to increase a girl's ethnic identity by having her learn more about African and African American culture.

Demonstrating the Lack of an African-Centered Framework

This is an activity that is best done at the beginning of a session/program prior to any lessons on Africa or African America. It demonstrates how African Americans are socialized to think of things that are non-African centered. Ask participants to name five Presidents. These could be president of a group, an organization, a country, a university, a company, etc. Have girls volunteer to call out the names of the Presidents taking turns. This exercise will show that the vast majority (if not all) of the participants will mostly name presidents who are not African or African American with the exception of President Barack Obama. It demonstrates that the immediate reaction is to not think of Presidents who are of African descent. When this first exercise is over, have girls name five nouns that are African American or of African descent. It could be five African American Presidents, five African American colleges and universities, five entertainers, etc. An alternative way to do this activity is to have girls call out the names of countries and African American women leaders.

Applying the Principles of Nguzo Saba

Another exercise is to have girls learn, discuss, and apply the Principles of Nguzo Saba (or the Principles of Kwanzaa). Kwanzaa is an African American celebration held between December 26 and 31 of each year. We have used the principles of Kwanzaa as a framework for discussing many topics. Kwanzaa was created by Dr. Maulana Karenga in 1966 to promote purpose, identity, and direction among Black people. The principles are universal and are relevant to other cultural groups. The principles can be discussed and learned in Swahili (the universal African language) and English. The seven principles follow. An eighth principle has been added to facilitate discussion on the importance of respect for self, parents, and others. For further information on Kwanzaa, see resource list for books written on Kwanza.

Umoja (Unity) – To strive for and maintain unity in the family, community, nation, and race.
Discussion Question: What is one thing that you can do to bring about unity within your family?
Kujichagulia (Self-Determination) – To define ourselves, name ourselves, create for ourselves, and speak for ourselves rather than to allow others to do these things for us.
Discussion Topic: Identify an African American woman who represents or who has spoken on behalf of African Americans?
Ujima (Collective work and responsibility) – To build and maintain our community together to make our sisters' and brothers' problems our problems and to solve them together.
Discussion Question: What can you do collectively to solve a problem within your school or community? Encourage girls to think of ways this can be done by working collectively.
Ujamaa (Cooperative Economics) – To build and maintain our own stores, shops, and other businesses and to profit from them together.
Discussion Question: Identify African American businesses in your community. How can you support these businesses?
Nia (Purpose) – To make our collective work the building and developing of our community in order to restore our people to their traditional greatness.

Discussion Question: Identify a project that can improve your community. How would you carry it out?

Kuumba (Creativity) – To do always as much as we can, in the way we can, in order to leave our community more beautiful and beneficial than when we inherited it.

Discussion Question: What is your talent? How can you use it to help your community?

Imani (faith) – To believe with all our heart in our people, our parents, our teachers, our leaders, and the righteousness and victory of our struggle.

Discussion Question: What does it mean to have faith?

Heshma (Respect) – to respect ourselves, our parents, and others.

Discussion Question: What are some of the ways in which you can show respect?

These principles can also be used to frame discussions around identity, relationships, and how to avoid problem behaviors. For example, Umoja can provide a starting framework in a discussion of the importance of the family and the community to how we feel about ourselves. We have used the principle of kujichagulia to introduce discussions about self-determination, and how it is up to each girl to take responsibility for her own health and well-being.

Expose Participants to Successful African American Female Adults

Invite African American female adults to talk about their careers or arrange for girls to spend time with a successful female adult. We have found that girls are most excited by women entrepreneurs, and we have invited African American female business owners to our sessions. These businesses have been both traditional (i.e., beauty shop owners) and nontraditional (president of computer-based and technology firms). We have also had students attending both predominately White and historically Black colleges and universities talk to our girls about their choices of college, their preparation for college, and what college life is like.

Discuss what it Means to be a Person of African Descent

Conversations can be held about what it means to be an African American. These conversations should begin by asking girls to vocalize what they think of when they think of (1) Africans and/or (2) African Americans. One girl told me that when she thought of African Americans she thought of violence and drugs. When I probed why, she said that this was all that she saw. When I pointed out that the neighborhood she lived in was all African American and that she was not exposed to people other than African Americans, she could began to see that her vision of African Americans was limited to her exposure to African Americans in her neighborhood and school. In the discussion, accept all impressions and descriptions. Let the girls figure out what is wrong with generalizing and stereotyping about African Americans and people of African descent.

To the extent feasible, introduce girls to other women of African descent who might come from Africa, the Caribbean, or a Latin American country. Many of our girls were surprised to find that people of African descent speak Spanish, French, and a host of other languages.

Promote Androgynous Gender Role Beliefs

The objective of these activities is to increase androgyny, which consists of both feminine/expressive and masculine/instrumental gender role beliefs.

Provide Opportunities for Expression of Both Masculine and Feminine Gender Role Beliefs

Provide opportunities for girls to participate in both nurturing/expressive and instrumental tasks. For example, have girls do community service projects that may be traditionally done by boys, such as building a ramp for people with disabilities or cleaning up a field by cutting the grass, and planting flowers and trees. At the same time, provide opportunities for girls to do caring tasks, such as fixing a meal for senior citizens and reading to younger children.

Discuss Career Options

As an activity, ask girls to list women who they are close to and to describe the career or employment situations of these women. Have them do the same for men. See if the girls can discern different patterns of career choices for males and females and discuss this. Have them discuss why they think these adults chose the careers they did. Encourage them to think about how things might differ now than when adults to whom they are close to chose their careers.

Promote Positive Relationships

The objective of these activities is to encourage girls to have positive relationships within their family and peer groups.

Identify and Discuss Positive Relationships

Ask girls to list or name different types of relationships they have. Using this list, have them discuss what these relationships mean to them. They are likely to discuss relationships with their mothers, fathers, siblings, and other family members.

Relationships with friends, boyfriends, and other romantic relationships may also be discussed.

Praise and Reward Girls when they are Doing Something Positive for Others

Look out for acts of kindness and concern girls show to others. This can be something as simple as letting another person take her turn, to helping a fellow student with her homework, to stopping negative comments or gossip. Because girls engage in relational aggression during this age, discourage gossip and exclusionary behavior by focusing on the positive.

One exercise we have done is to have the girls themselves select a person to win a "sister" prize each week/session. Criteria should be developed and agreed upon by the girls as to what constitutes the behavior for the sister prize. A variation of this activity is to have girls put a name of a person into a "sister box" when the person is seen doing a good deed. One name is pulled from the box each week.

Promote Positive Body Image

The objective of these activities is to promote positive body image and feelings of comfort about the body.

Analyze Media Messages

Provide a video clip and/or pictures from magazines of African American adolescent females. Have girls critically evaluate what is happening regarding the African American character. What does she look like? Why is she portrayed the way she is? What are positive and negative things about her? What would happen if these images are seen continually? Encourage girls to become media critics.

Resources

Belgrave, F.Z., Rawls, V., Butler, D., & Townsend, T. (2008). Sisters of Nia: A Cultural Curriculum to Empower African American Girls. Champaign, IL: Research.

Karenga, M. (1996). Kwanzaa: A Celebration of Family, Community and Culture. Los Angeles: University of Sankore Press.

Dr. Maulana Karenga, Creator of Kwanza, The Official Kwanazaa Website, http://www.officialkwanzaawebsite.org/index.shtml#Welcome (Retrieved 6/24/08).

Smart Girls (1998). Smart Girls: Skills Mastery and Resistance Training: A Small Group Program for Early Adolescent Girls for Ages 10 to 14. Boys and Girls Clubs of America.

Part II

Chapter 3
Family and Kin

> *"My mother, my grandmother, and my sisters. Because I see how they support themselves and they don't need any man to support them. They have their own jobs, they raising their own kids, basically and raising them successfully and teaching them what they need to know what they didn't learn when they were young ... my sisters teach their daughters not to think about boys at this age. The mistakes they made when they were thinking about boys and running around after them and how they got themselves in trouble and they never got to finish their education and they still manage to get a good job. They lead their daughters to know that boys are not important; you need to finish your high school education and then think about boys. Or finish your education first and then think about boys."*
>
> *13-year-old girl responding to the question, "who is important in your life?"*

The above quote shows the strong influence of mothers and other maternal relations on adolescent girls. Mothers ensure that their daughters learn the life skills and lessons necessary to navigate life. Girls learn from their parents how to care for others, do well in school, and how to be good citizens. African American girls' behaviors, beliefs, and attitudes are shaped by mothers and other members of her family more so than any other person or institution.

Socialization within the family begins at birth. Generally, the mother is the primary person responsible for her daughter's socialization. Others including fathers, grandmothers, and other family members may also assume this responsibility. Siblings and other relatives, including aunts, uncles, and cousins, are similarly influential in the lives of African American girls. Throughout the chapter, research and literature on the role the family plays in supporting the healthy psychosocial development of African American girls is highlighted. As will be discussed, her family is the primary agent for shaping who she is and who she will become.

This chapter begins with an overview of the African American family. A discussion of family structure and well-being and girls' roles within their families follows. Relationships with mothers and fathers influence girls and relationships and communication patterns with mothers and fathers are discussed next, followed by a discussion of family supervision and monitoring. The "Recommendations

F.Z. Belgrave, *African American Girls*, Advancing Responsible Adolescent Development, 33
DOI 10.1007/978-1-4419-0090-6_3, © Springer Science+Business Media, LLC 2009

and Resources" section of this chapter provides activities on strengthening family cohesion, relationships, and parental effectiveness.

The African American Family

Robert Hill (1998) defined the African American family as a household related by blood or marriage or function that provides basic instrumental and expressive functions to its members. By instrumental functions, he meant that the family takes care of the physical, material, and safety needs of its members. Food, clothing, shelter, education, and health care are examples of instrumental needs. Expressive needs are those that have to do with love, support, nurturance, and connections to others. Examples of expressive needs are having someone to talk to, someone to confine in, and someone to ask for support and advice.

Who is in her Family?

African American families are diverse and there is no one typical African American family. At the same time, there are some characteristics of many African American families. African America families are often multigenerational. Three or even four generations, including children, parents, and grandparents, may live in the same household. The African American family can also be described as "extended." Members other than the immediate and biological members of the family such as mother, father, and children feel and act like family members. Extended family members may live within or outside the home and include grandparents, cousins, aunts, and uncles. It is also not uncommon to find cousins living together, and these cousins may feel and act like siblings. Sometimes people who are not related biologically or by adoption are members of the extended family. Sociologists refer to these individuals as fictive kin. Fictive kin feel and behave like members of the family. These individuals are sometimes called "big mama," "play sister," "play brother," etc. Having an extended and intergenerational family means that African American girls may have several significant adults to whom she feels connected to and who are available to supervise and monitor her behavior.

Most African American girls live in households without a father present. The 2006 American Community Survey provides data on the family structure of African American teens between the ages of 15 and 19. About 35.2% live in married-couple households, 54.4% live in mother-headed households with no husband present, 7.5% live in father-headed households with no wife present, and 2.9% live in nonfamily households (U.S. Census Bureau, 2006 American Community Survey). Thus African American girls are most likely to live in households without fathers present.

Grandparents

African American grandparents are also often a part of the African American house-hold. About 20% of African American grandparents reside in households with their children and grandchildren. Grandmother's presence is seen across socioeconomic levels and conditions. For example, Michele Obama's mother, Marian Robinson, moved into the White House to help care for the two Obama girls. In about 11% of grandparent-present households, grandparents are responsible for the care of at least one grandchild (U.S. Census, 2004). Grandmothers help in managing the household and the children's activities. Grandparents may also provide firm but loving discipline. It may be the grandmother who establishes and or reinforces routines and rituals for meals, religious participation, and other activities within the home. In our discussions with girls who have been involved in our programs and research, many report that they feel close to and attached to their grandmothers. In fact, the teen's grandmother is often the adult who assists with rearing a teen mother's child.

Family Structure and Well-Being

Family structure has to do with what does the family look like. An example of a "typical" family in the United States might be a husband, wife, and two children. However, for an African American girl, a "typical" family might be two children with a single female parent. Because single-parent households tend to be poorer and in less desirable neighborhoods, research has generally reported a negative impact of single-parent status on children's outcome (Alexander, 1997; Smith, Brooks-Gunn, & Klebanov, 2000).

Researchers have reported unfavorable academic, social, psychological, and behavioral consequences of children from single-parent households. Some of these include earlier school dropout, earlier and more risky sexual behavior, greater juvenile delinquency, more drug use, etc. (Hollist & McBroom, 2006; Steinberg, 1987). However, when family income is taken into consideration, children from single-parent households may not fare any worse than those in two-parent households. For example, using national survey data, Biblarz and Raftery (1999) found no negative effects for children raised in single-parent households when mother's education and occupation were considered.

Another study by Ricciuti (2004) showed that children raised in households with different family structures did not differ academically. In a study that followed students for several years (from ages 6–7 to 12–13), Ricciuti (2004) used a national data set to determine if single parenthood for 6- and 7-year olds had adverse cognitive and social effects 6 years later when these children reached 12–13 years of age. Three types of family groups were identified: (1) single parent; (2) two parent; and (3) a change group (change from two to one parent or vice versa). The sample consisted of African American, White, and Latino children. Ricciuti found no relationship between family group and children's achievement test scores or problem behavior scores during the years between 6–7 and 12–13. The author noted that the potential adverse consequences of single parenthood for children may be reduced by other characteristics that support positive parenting for children.

In overview, research concerning growing up in a single-parent household is equivocal, with some studies reporting harmful effects and others reporting no detrimental effects. What does seem to matter with regard to children's psychological and social functioning is whether resources are available for single-parent-headed households (Alexander, 1997). Poverty is more likely to exist within single-parent-headed households (than two-parent households), and poverty accounts for some of the poorer outcomes often associated with being raised in a single-parent-headed household. Being raised in a single-parent household is not an automatic precursor to high-risk sexual behavior (Cunningham & Thornton, 2007). This is especially so if support is provided by other adults. The presence of another caring family member, which is often a grandparent, aunt, or uncle, can decrease parental burden by assisting with childcare, monetary aid, and guidance for teen girls (Chiteji & Hamilton, 2005).

Raising Girls in African American Households

Parenting African American girls presents both unique opportunities and challenges. Issues that African American girls face that African American males and girls from other racial and ethnic groups do not face include sexism, racism, and sometimes classism. These "isms" can make for a hostile environment for African American girls growing up in this country. Racism and sexism can be very subtle, yet the pervasive and the institutional nature of racism and sexism affect life-course expectations and subsequent achievement if not addressed within the family.

Even some religious institutions, central in the lives of many African American families, convey sexism through the restrictive roles females hold within these institutions. Women including those who have been trained as ministers are not usually the leaders in the African American Protestant Churches, the denomination to which the majority of African Americans belong (Cook & Wiley, 2000). Women's responsibilities are more likely in service and helping, i.e., mission, hospitability, and secretarial and administrative activities. When sexism and racism are coupled with classism, there is even greater potential for girls to have poor life-course expectations and achievement. While these "isms" are fairly institutionalized in this country, they can certainly be challenged by well-informed parents. One way in which racism and sexism can be addressed is through racial and gender socialization.

Racial and Gender Socialization

Racial socialization is the process by which parents socialize their children how to live in this society. When parents socialize their children about race they become aware of their race and of themselves as Black or African American (Boykin & Toms, 1985; Thornton, 1997). Racial socialization teaches problem-solving skills so that children can solve race-related problems (Coard & Sellers, 2005). Racial socialization increases racial identity, self-esteem, and competence.

There are three types of racial socialization messages African American parents use to socialize their daughters (Boykin & Toms, 1985; Thornton, 1997). One message is that they must participate in the majority American culture. This socialization message encourages girls to go to school and to get good grades so that they can go to college. Parents of daughters might also emphasize roles and responsibilities of women in this society. For example, girls might be socialized to only date one boy at a time, to learn how to do of household chores, and to be able to financially take care of themselves. These types of gender socialization messages likely contribute to androgynous gender role beliefs among African American girls.

Another type of message that parents provide to their children is to prepare them for being a minority in an environment that might not be accepting of minorities. These types of messages socialize the child about what they would need to do well in this society because of being African American and female. These messages might have parents encouraging their daughters to focus on school and not boys to reduce the likelihood that their education will be shortchanged. They might tell their daughters that it is more difficult for African American than White girls to succeed in this society. A common saying is "you have to be twice as good to get one half as far." A third type of socialization message is to teach children to value and to honor their African American heritage. Parents might, for example, talk to their daughters about historical African American women and the contributions of these women. They might also tell her about strong women in their families who have overcome obstacles.

Racial and gender socialization messages contribute to positive socialization experiences of African American girls (Coard & Sellers, 2005). Girls whose parents use different types of socialization messages are likely to fare better than those who only use one type of message. For example, focusing on the mainstream message about the importance of education while excluding messages about how to live as an African American girl may obscure how to optimally function as an African American in this country. Socialization messages about race and gender likely protect/buffer girls from stressors arising from sexism and racism as these messages help girls learn to cope with racism and sexism (Bynum, Burton, & Best, 2007).

Parenting Methods

Methods parents use for disciplining and monitoring their daughters vary. African American parents are more likely than parents from other ethnic groups to use physical punishment to discipline their children (Bradley, 1998). Growing up in this country requires African American children to know that there are limits on their behavior. Physical punishment while seemingly harsh may provide an instant message that some behavior is unacceptable and must be stopped immediately. Physical punishment of African American children generally stops (although not always) when they reach early adolescence especially among girls.

Although many African American parents use physical punishment while disciplining younger children there is a great deal of variability (Bradley, 1998). Other types of disciplines include restriction of activities and possessions as well as verbal reprimands. African American parents especially mothers often give the message that they are loved even when disciplining. Girls whose parents use a combination of both warmth and discipline seem to do well (Lansford, Deater-Deckard, Dodge & Bates, 2004; Magnus & Cowen, 1999). Having girls assume responsibilities within the household are other ways in which African American teen girls are kept in check and monitored.

African American Girls' Roles within the Family

Many African American girls are responsible for family and household chores, including cleaning, cooking, doing laundry, and taking care of younger siblings. Sibling child-care responsibilities begin during pre- and early adolescence at about the ages of 11 and 12, although in some families even younger girls are expected to care for their younger siblings. Girls may be responsible for preparing their younger siblings' meals, supervising his or her play, taking the child to and from school or day care, supervising baths, and in general supervising the daily activities of the younger child.

Child-care responsibilities for siblings can be both beneficial and detrimental to girls' growth and development. Caring for a younger sibling promotes responsibility and the development of life skills that can be useful in other life domains. Teen girls who care for younger siblings contribute to the household (i.e., money is saved in child-care expenses). Finally, taking care of younger sibling structures the teen's activities and time while she is not at school. On the other hand, too many child-care responsibilities can interfere with social and academic activities that could also be beneficial. An intervention program recognized the responsibilities African American girls had in the rearing of their siblings and is discussed next.

Project Naja

The high prevalence of girls with sibling child-care responsibilities presented a problem in a community-based intervention program I evaluated (Belgrave, Chase-Vaughn, Gray, Dixon-Addison, & Cherry, 2000). Many girls were not able to participate in this after-school intervention because of child-care responsibilities. The program, called Project Naja, was designed to help African American teen girls aged 10–14 improve along dimensions such as self-esteem, healthy values, racial identity, and positive peer relations. However, in our initial contact with girls and their families, we found that many of these girls could not participate because they were responsible for taking care of one or more younger siblings after school. This typically involved picking younger siblings up after day care or school, walking them home, and watching them until their parents came home. In order to enroll girls in our program, we had to also provide a program for their younger siblings. We partnered with a local Head Start and identified both girls in the targeted age range and their younger siblings for this program. The program achieved its objectives with regard to increasing self-concept, ethnic identity, and other positive attributes among program participants (Belgrave, Brome, & Hampton, 2000). Many of the teen girls would not have been able to participate in the program if they could not bring their younger siblings with them.

Mother–Daughter Relationships and Communication

A girl's relationship and communication with her mother is very influential to her well-being and development. Communication involves sending, receiving, and understanding each other's messages. If there are problems in any of these steps, communication suffers. The majority of the girls in our studies and programs have reported positive relationships with their mothers. Although there were some exceptions, in general, girls reported that they admired and had learned much from their mothers.

Mothers teach and socialize their daughters about every aspect of her life, including being female, being a mother, how to relate to and care for others, and about health, and sexuality. They also teach her what it takes to make a good living in this country, and how to reach economic and career success. As discussed in the previous chapter, mothers teach their daughters how to be both independent and nurturing. However, not all African American mother–daughter relationships are positive, and there is sometimes conflict.

Conflict may arise during early adolescence when girls began to seek autonomy and the right to make their own decisions (Costigan, Cauce, & Etchison, 2007). Her need to be autonomous may create stress and conflict in the mother–daughter relationship. However, conflict is not always bad. In a study of African American adolescent girls and their mothers, Costigan, Cauce, & Etchison (2007) found that greater adolescent decision-making autonomy at Time 1 led to greater self-esteem at a later point in time. The authors speculate that the ability of mothers and daughters to recognize areas of disagreement may work well for girls in the long run. Conflict between mothers and daughters can be beneficial if families are able to resolve this conflict.

Mothers influence their daughter's directly and indirectly. Directly, mothers communicate with and talk to their daughters. Indirectly, they model to their daughters, ways in which to behave. For example daughters with mothers who had children at a young age are more likely to have children at a young age themselves. Mothers who have high levels of education expect their daughters to have high levels of education, and this is what generally happens.

What do African American Girls Learn from their Mothers?

African American mothers communicate both verbally and nonverbally what it means to be an African American woman in this country. As discussed in the previous chapter, mothers socialize daughters to be assertive and independent while at the same time to be caring and nurturing. These daughters become androgynous and have both masculine traits like independence and assertiveness and feminine traits like nurturance, compassion, and warmth. Historically, African American women have had to be breadwinners, and to assume responsibility for caring for their families and others because of limited opportunities for African American males. Girls observe the dual identity of their mothers and other significant women in their lives and internalize these identities (Ashcraft & Belgrave, 2004).

Not all girls are exposed to positive role models from mothers. Some girls are exposed to deleterious behaviors from mothers and significant other females. For example, mothers and other significant women may convey that it is ok to be in dysfunctional relationships, use drugs, and be financially irresponsible. Mothers may also model poor partner choices when they remain in dysfunctional and abusive relationships.

When Mothers Model Poor Partner Choices

The fact is that African American women expect to and are more likely to be single than African American males and women from other ethnic groups. There are many factors contributing to African American women's singleness, including incarceration and educational status of African American men. Limited partner options may contribute to African American females tolerating unhealthy relationships with male partners. These relationships may include relationships with males who are abusive and/or with males who do not contribute financially, socially, or emotionally to the care of the children or household. Mothers also model what is expected of women in order to "keep the peace" or to keep a man. In interviews with 15 African American teen girls and their mothers, Ashcraft and Belgrave (2004) noted that several girls reported poor relationship choices of their mothers. Some of the girls reported that their mothers were abused physically and verbally by male partners.

Other mothers in the Ashcraft study modeled to their daughters that the way in which men show that they care for them is when they provide them with material things such as clothing, trips to the hair-and-nail salon, and entertainment. The high value placed on material possessions was likely linked to the limited resources of girls and their families since they resided in low-resource communities. Having a male partner pay for getting her hair and nails done or buying her a new outfit may seem like evidence of affection and care to these girls. At the same time, many of the girls did not articulate that what was important in a relationship were values of trust, respect, and open communication. This behavior excuses men from providing social or emotional support. The findings from the Ashcraft study suggest that mothers especially those in poor households and communities may need to be cognizant of how gifts from boys and men can come to be associated with caring and being a good partner without consideration of other personal attributes (i.e., kindness, respect, mutuality, etc.).

In summary, mothers have a tremendous influence on their daughters and daughters learn from their mothers' core values, beliefs, expectations, and ways to behave. Mothers can model both positive and negative behaviors especially in regard to relationships.

Father–Daughter Relationships and Communication

Mothers and fathers influence their daughter in both similar and unique ways. While there has been less written about father–daughter relationships especially among African American girls, we know that father–daughter relationships and communications affect all aspects of her life. Fathers may be especially influential in the development of their daughter's image of herself.

What do African American Girls Relationships with their Fathers Look Like?

Interviews with African American and Latina girls in early adolescence addressed this question (Way and Gillman, 2000). Girls from low-income homes were asked questions about their relationships with their fathers. Way and Gillman identified four themes by which girls described their relationships with their fathers.

The first theme addressed ways in which adolescent girls spent time with and communicated with their fathers. The girls tended to talk about the activities they did together with their fathers such as playing sports, attending athletic events, and going to amusement parks. Girls preferred to discuss intimate topics with their mothers and not with their fathers.

Girls were not less engaged with their fathers than with their mothers, but they were engaged in different ways. Girls engaged with their fathers by doing things with them or sharing activities. The girls enjoyed this type of relationship. This pattern of relationship was seen irrespective of whether the fathers lived in the household.

The second theme was that girls wanted to spend more time than they currently spent with their fathers. They wanted to share more activities with their fathers. This included talking about sports, the world, and school. The third theme was on girls' thoughts about their fathers' protection of them from the dangers of the world. Fathers tended to become more protective of their daughters as they grew older. Fathers were concerned about the potential problems arising from relationships with boys. These types of concerns often led to arguments as daughters typically wanted more freedom than fathers wanted to give. Although some of the girls understood why their father was protective, they also felt that his overprotectiveness interfered with her ability to grow. While fathers tended to be protective of their daughters, daughters also felt the same way about their fathers. The fourth theme from the interviews by Way and Gillman addressed daughters' protectiveness of their fathers. These girls indicated that they took their fathers' side in family arguments. Some of the girls wanted to live with their fathers, even those who may have had a history of abuse or neglectful behavior.

One way in which fathers connect with their daughters is through sports, and sports may be a means in which fathers communicate with their daughters. Fathers may encourage daughters to participate in organized sports, or they may simply watch a sporting events together (Kellar-DeMers, 2001). Research suggests that sports not only contributes to positive father–daughter relationships but is also a protective factor for other problem behaviors. Studies have found that girls' participation in organized sports is related to decreases in sexual activity and other high-risk behaviors (Kulig, Brenner, & McManus, 2003; McNulty-Eitle & Eitle, 2002).

Fathers become less involved as daughters mature physically. Puberty has been linked to decreased involvement of fathers in their daughters' lives. Hill (1998) found among seventh grade girls that both fathers and mothers reported lower involvement with daughters who had began to menstruate within the past 6 months than those who were premenarcheal.

Influence of Fathers on Daughter's Self-Attributes

Father–daughter relationships are important in the shaping of a daughter's body image, self-worth, and other self-attributes. A positive relationship with her father may be especially beneficial during the period of early adolescence when girls become aware of their changing bodies and how boys respond to those changes. The media contributes to her body awareness, and this media exposure often results in a more negative evaluation of her body and her sexual attractiveness. Fathers can play a role in buffering daughter's perception of self in light of unrealistic media images (Graber & Sontag, 2006).

Dixon, Gill, and Adair (2003) administered surveys to the fathers of 103 girls (ages: 13–15) and asked them their beliefs about the importance of physical appearance, slimness, and weight control. Their daughters completed a survey about eating habits and diet beliefs. Positive associations were found between the father's belief in the importance of physical attractiveness and their daughter's dieting behavior. In a study of African American girls in early adolescence, Hedgepeth (2008) found that more positive father–daughter relationships were associated with more positive body image satisfaction and lower image acculturation. Those girls who had a more positive relationship with their father were more likely to value aspects of their physical appearance that was more Africentric (as opposed to Eurocentric). The finding from the Hedgepeth study suggests that girls who feel accepted by their fathers for how they look are not as likely to seek other external standards for defining their beauty.

In terms of self-esteem, fathers may have an even greater impact than mothers on their daughter's self-esteem. A study by Richards, Gitelson, Petersen, & Hurtig (1991) found that there is a more powerful relationship between fathers and daughters' self-esteem such that daughters' self-esteem appeared to be improved by their positive experiences with their fathers more so than their mothers. Other researchers have found that when a daughter feels positive affirmations from her father, she has higher self-esteem and also less fear of intimacy (Scheffler & Naus, 1999).

The influence of fathers' relationships on their daughters' self-worth seems to be independent of the girls' relationship with their mother. Amato (1994) found that regardless of the quality of the mother–child relationship, a daughter's closeness to her father was significantly associated with her being happier, more satisfied, and less distressed. In another study, daughters displayed more helping behavior when they perceived more opportunities, were more involved, and perceived more reinforcement with their fathers. In this study, the daughter's behavior was not directly influenced by their mothers (Kosterman, Haggerty, Spoth, & Redmond, 2004).

Father–Daughter Communication and Conflict

Fathers and daughters may communicate differently when fathers are alone with their daughters than when they are not. Smetana, Abernethy, and Harris (2000) investigated change over time and contextual differences in middle-class African American adolescent–parent relationships. Dyadic and triadic family interactions were observed. When comparing dyadic and triadic contexts, the findings revealed that fathers engaged in more positive communication, and adolescents were more receptive to fathers when they interacted alone as opposed to when the mother was present. Fathers seemed to communicate more effectively, and adolescents were more willing to listen to fathers' message when mothers were absent. Furthermore, adolescents' communications with fathers became more positive over time only in the father–adolescent dyadic context. The authors suggest that father–adolescent interactions may represent a positive and crucial context for adolescent development.

In a study of over 300 low-income African American adolescent girls, Coley (2003) investigated the relationship between father–daughter conflict (anger and alienation) and girls' emotional well-being. The author found that daughters' anger and alienation from fathers were related to greater emotional and behavioral problems. When there was both low contact and high levels of anger in the father–daughter relationship there were particularly deleterious psychosocial outcomes for adolescent girls.

Father–Daughter Relationships and Sexual Behavior

The relationship that a girl has with her father is likely to influence her sexual attitudes and behaviors. Fathers are important in conveying positive relationship choices given that often media images of male–female relationships are sexually exploitative in nature. Fathers can model nonsexual interactions with the opposite sex. Girls tend to initiate sexual activity at a later age when fathers communicate disapproval of sexual activity (Dittus, Jaccard, & Gordon, 1997). In the study by Dittus and colleagues, the authors found a lower age of sexual initiation for both African American males and females when fathers had communicated disapproval of sexual activity. Father disapproval of premarital sex was also correlated with current sexual activity. Additionally, the authors found that girls who lived in the households with their fathers were less likely to have initiated sex than those who did not live with their fathers. Perhaps girls who live with their fathers have more opportunities to discuss sexual topics.

Harris-Peterson (2006) interviewed African American females in late adolescence about father–daughter sexual communication, specifically the type and amount of sexual behavior messages delivered by their fathers. Interviews conveyed three themes. Fathers were directive, insightful, and/or absent/avoidant. Directive fathers discussed topics such as sexual protection in a clear manner and also provided messages about social norms and expectations, making clear what their preferences were for their daughter's sexual behavior. Insightful fathers were likely to engage their daughters in on-going conversations about romantic and sexual relations, and to discuss their daughter's current romantic relationships. These fathers also discussed the emotional aspects that occur with sexual relationships. Lastly, absent/avoidant fathers did not discuss sex with their daughters and deferred such communication to mothers. Directive and insightful fathers had the most positive influence on their daughter's sexual development. Women with directive and insightful fathers believed that their fathers influenced their sexual choices by delivering messages concerning what to expect when dating and by modeling appropriate male behavior. The daughters of absent fathers reported feeling rejection, regret, and pain at the lack of a closer relationship.

In summary, girls interact with and have different types of relationships with their fathers than their mothers. When girls reach puberty, relationships and communications with parents may be disrupted. Yet, this is a period in her life in which positive relationships and communication are very crucial. Parental monitoring also is important and will be discussed next.

Parental Monitoring and Structure

Parental monitoring is another contributing factor to adolescent girl's well-being. Parenting monitoring is the extent to which parents are aware of their child's activities and whereabouts outside school (Crosby, DiClemente, Wingood, Long, &

Harrington, 2003). Monitoring involves supervising activities such as homework, activities with friends, and other structured and unstructured extracurricular activities. Girls who live in households where there is monitoring will fare much better than those who live in households in which they are not monitored and supervised.

Monitoring is a deterrent to sexual activity and other risky behaviors as shown by the results of a survey of approximately 2,000 African American males and females from urban high schools (Cohen, Farley, Taylor, Martin, & Schuster, 2002). Of those who were having sexual activity, 56% reported that it occurred on a week day. Furthermore, sexual activity took place usually in a home setting, either their home, their partner's, or a friend's home. These activities usually took place after school. The majority of these incidences occurred prior to 6 p.m. There was no difference in supervision for teens in one- and two-parent families (Cohen et al., 2002).

In fact, parental monitoring has been cited as an effective strategy for teen pregnancy prevention. In a study of 360 adolescents of whom about 36% were African American, researchers found that an average of 3 hours a day of unsupervised time with peers was associated with an increase in sexual activity (Borawaski, Ievers-Landis, Lovereen, & Trapl, 2003). Another study found that adolescent girls who reported less parental monitoring were almost twice as likely to contract sexually transmitted infections as those who reported more frequent parental monitoring (Crosby et al., 2003).

African American parents of lower socioeconomic status may be more restrictive in their monitoring of girls than those of higher socioeconomic status. Evidence of earlier and risky sexual behavior such as teen pregnancy and parenting may account for higher monitoring. There is also more neighborhood risk for violence among girls from lower socioeconomic communities (Garcia-Coll, Meyer, & Brillon, 1995; Parke & Buriel, 1998). In a study, Way and Gillman (2000) reported that parental restrictiveness was one problem voiced by urban girls from a lower socioeconomic community. These adolescents whose ages ranged from 12 to 13 reported that their fathers were protective and wanted to guard them against the dangers of the world. This protection included prohibiting certain activities, warning about the dangers of not following the rules, and giving advice about boys (Way and Gillman, 2000). On the other hand, in a study of two-parent, middle-class African American parents, Smetana and Chuang (2001) found that negotiation and reasoning were often-used parenting strategies. But even so fathers of these girls were still likely to define firm discipline as nonnegotiable in specific areas such as homework and curfew.

Parental Influences on Daughter's Life-Course Expectations

A girl's conceptualization of who she is and who she can become is influenced by her parents and other kin. Her career and education attainment and expectations are heavily influenced by her mother. In one study of African American teens, researchers found that a mother's expectation of whether she would attend college was the most important predictor of the daughter's educational expectations (McLoyd & Hernandez-Jozefowicz, 1996).

Mother's education is correlated with her daughter's actual academic outcomes. Educated mothers are more likely to have values that encourage their daughters to do well academically. This is not to say that daughters with mothers who do not have high levels of education will not do well. Sometimes, the opposite effect occurs for mothers with low levels of education. These mothers, wanting their daughter to have greater life choices than they had, encourage their daughters to get an education.

Summary

We have seen in this chapter the critical role that parents and family play in shaping their daughter's lives and in helping her through a successful adolescent transition. African American families are diverse and there is no one typical African American family. African America families are often multigenerational and extended, and may include grandparents. The majority of African American girls live in single-female-headed households. A girl's relationship and communication with her mother is very influential to her well-being and development, and mothers have a tremendous influence on their daughters. Mothers model both positive and negative behaviors sometimes negative relationship choices are modeled. Fathers also influence their daughters in many important domains, including body image, self-worth, and sexual behavior. Communication and activities with fathers decrease as the girls get older. Parenting monitoring and supervision are important to the well-being of girls, and girls who are not monitored and supervised are at higher risk for sexual activity especially during the after-school period.

Recommendations and Resources

The following suggestions and recommendations can be implemented within single-family settings/and or within group settings such as family, after school programs, churches, community and recreational centers, etc.

Monitor and Supervise

The first recommendation is perhaps the most essential and involves monitoring and supervision. Daughters should be taught to be responsible for letting parents know where they are at all times. The 2–3 hours period after school is often the prime time for lack of supervision. Participation in structured after-school activities helps in this regard. Having girls volunteer at a local library, recreational center, or the like are activities that will structure after school time.

Encourage and Provide Opportunities for Meaningful Relationships with Males

As discussed, male parental figures are important for several reasons. Fathers are role models for the kind of men their daughter eventually chooses. Girls who grow up with absentee fathers or fathers who do not interact with them are often more in need of male attention. If fathers do not provide this attention, it might be gained from an undesirable male partner. If daughters do not have an involved father, connections with male grandfathers, uncles, brothers, etc. are important. Many fathers are more involved in their daughters' lives when she is young and began to disconnect as she grows older. Plan activities that can be shared by girls and their fathers at all age levels.

Communication is Essential

Without communication there is no relationship. Listening is the most important skill a parent can have. If her behavior is not appropriate, comment on the behavior and not her as a person. Use time spent in the car and other down time periods to broach subjects and topics to get an idea of what is going on in her world. Listen to what she and her friends talk about. Shared activities are good ways to increase bonding and affection. This can be routine activities such as watching a television program or a movie together, working on household chores, or taking a walk. Also, parents should schedule time for special activities with their daughters. These can be gender related such as getting nails done, doing hair, or cooking a meal. Be aware of scheduling barriers to shared activities, so set up a routine where these activities can be done within the natural context of day-to-day activities. Family meals are also important. Make sure that the family has at least some meals together on a regular basis. Engage daughters' help in preparing the meals.

Parents Should Racially Socialize their Daughters about what it Means to be an African American Girl and Woman

Racial socialization involves parents talking to their daughter about their race and about how to survive and thrive in this country as an African American and also as a woman. This involves socialization to the main culture as well as to African American culture. Parents can talk to their daughters about how things were for African Americans and women in their generation and what she needs to do to be a successful African American woman. Parents may want to patronize African American-owned female businesses with their daughter that are both traditionally female (e.g., beauty salons) and nontraditional (e.g., construction sites). Parents may also discuss positive African American role models in politics, business, arts, and entertainment. Conversely, they can discuss public figures who are not positive role models.

Have Girls Reflect on what Family Means to them

One suggested group activity is to have discussions among two groups of girls. In one group, girls could identify ways in which they are like their mother (or another significant female adult), and in the other group girls could identify ways in which they are like their father (or another significant male adult). Each group could develop a list to see and present this list to the larger group. The larger group could discuss how the traits identified for maternal and paternal figures differ.

Another group activity is to have girls write an essay about influential female family members in their lives (other than their mother or mother figure). Family can include biological family or persons that feel like family to the girl (fictive kin). Each girl can do a 2–3 min presentation on the influence this individual has had on her life.

Evidence-Based Parenting Programs

There are a number of parenting programs that can be used to increase effective parenting effectiveness, family cohesion, and to improve teen–parent communication. These programs also improve adolescent psychosocial outcomes such as increased self-esteem, life skills, and reduced drug use. The three programs discussed next have been evaluated and have demonstrated effectiveness with African American families and adolescents.

The *Effective Black Parenting Program* (EBPP) is a culturally relevant parenting, skill-building program that attends to the unique history, values, and life circumstances of African Americans. The EBPP, created to address the needs of Black children, was designed to assist educators, organizations, child-care providers, and parents in raising competent and achieving Black children (Alvy, 1994). The EBPP can be used with families of children of all ages. The program fosters effective family communication, healthy Black identity, extended family values, child growth and development, and healthy self-esteem. The EBPP has 14 three-hour sessions and a graduation ceremony. The curriculum covers culturally specific parenting strategies, general parenting strategies, parenting skills, and special program topics such as single parenting and preventing substance use. The program can be implemented in a variety of settings, including schools, recreational facilities, churches, social service agencies, etc. The program is usually implemented in small groups of parents (8–20). There have been several published papers on the success of the program, and participants in the program improve in positive parenting practices, relationships, and communication. The book *Parent Training Today: A Social Necessity*

(Alvy, 1994) summarizes findings from the development of this program. For further information contact, Keby Alvy, Center for the Improvement of Child Caring, 11331 Ventura Boulevard, Suite 103, Studio City, CA 91604-3147, (818) 980-0903 or (800) 325-2422 or visit this website: *www.ciccparenting.org*

Creating Lasting Family Connections (CLFC) is a comprehensive family strengthening, substance abuse, and violence prevention curriculum that has shown that youth and families in high-risk environments can be assisted to become strong, healthy, and supportive people (see Council on Prevention and Education of Substances/*http://copes.org*). CLFC has been used with families of children aged 9–17 and with African American and other ethnic minority families. Skills learned in the CLFC program protect parents and children against environmental risk factors by teaching appropriate skills for personal growth, family enhancement, and interpersonal communication. CLFC can be implemented within community agencies such as churches, schools, recreation centers, and court-referred settings. The program consists of six training modules.

Findings from an evaluation of the CLFC show significant increases in family bonding and communication, use of community services, children's ability to resist drugs, and a reduction in the use of alcohol and other drugs. More information on the program can be obtained by visiting the CLFC website and/or by contacting Ted Strader, Ph.D., Council on Prevention and Education, Substances, Inc. (502) 583–6820 Web site: www.copes.org/include/clfc.htm

The Strengthening Families Program for Parents and Youth 10–14 (SFP 10 = 14) is a video-based program designed to reduce adolescent substance abuse and other problem behaviors among youth 10–14 years old. This program has been successfully used with ethnic minority families, including African American families. The SFP is delivered within parent, youth, and family sessions using narrated videos that portray typical youth-and-parent situations. Interactive sessions include role playing, discussions, learning games, and family projects. The program improves parenting skills, develops life skills in youth, and strengthens family bonds. The basic program is implemented over a 7-week period and is delivered usually in the evenings and involves both parents and youth. The SFP has been effective at building parent skills (e.g., monitoring, setting limits, and expressing affection) and youth skills (e.g., resisting peer pressure, making positive goals, and managing strong emotions) and changing behavior. For further information contact, Catherine Webb, Iowa State University Extension, Institute for Social and Behavioral Research, Iowa State University, Ames, IA 50010, (515) 294–1426 or view web site at: www.extension.iastate.edu/sfp/

Resources

Institute for the Advanced Study of Black Families. This Center, directed by Dr. Wade Nobles has as its stated mission the reunification of the Black family, the reclamation of Black culture, and the revitalization of the Black community. It accomplishes this through research, education, and training. See website for further information http://www.iasbflc.org/mission.htmThddre

McLoyd, V. C., Hill, N. E., & Dodge, K. A. (2005). *African American Family Life. African American Families*. New York: Guildford. This edited volume presents a comprehensive overview of the challenges and opportunities facing parents, children, and communities. It also discusses health and key cultural and social processes.

Substance Abuse and Mental Health Administration, National Registry of Evidence Based Programs http://www.nrepp.samhsa.gov/find.asp. This registry includes information on over 100 interventions to prevent problem behaviors. It identifies programs that can be used specifically with African Americans, females, and families.

Chapter 4
Peers and Friends

"...my relationship with girls is different from boys because girls like to gossip a lot and keep stuff going – they'll come to you and tell you something, then they'll go back and tell the next person and tell them that, and they just like to gossip and keep things going ... they can't hold secrets unless the female is your family ... Boys, some of them gossip but not a lot of them."

13-year-old girl's response to question, "how are relationships with boys different than relationships with girls?"

Outside the family, girls spend more time with friends than with any other individuals. Our friendship and peer group are often a reflection of who we are. During adolescence, girls select (or are selected by) friends. For the most part, girls choose to be with friends and peers who are similar socioeconomically and who hold the same values and beliefs, although there are some exceptions with African American girls. In this chapter, the nature of friendship among African American girls and the influence of friends and peers on their well-being are examined. The chapter discusses how friends and peers influence attitudes and behaviors both positively and negatively. This chapter begins with definitions followed by a discussion of why friendships are so important to African American girls.

Definitions

Definitions of friends, peers, cliques, and gangs are provided by the Merriam-Webster online dictionary. A friend is a person whom we are attached to by affection or esteem. A peer is a person who belongs to the same societal group based on age, grade, or status. A clique is a narrow exclusive circle or group of friends who may be held together by common interests. A gang is defined as a group of persons working to unlawful or antisocial ends, such as a band of antisocial adolescents. What is common to all these terms is the element of connection to and relationships with others. As discussed in Chapter 2, the relational nature of girls makes friends and peers especially important.

F.Z. Belgrave, *African American Girls*, Advancing Responsible Adolescent Development, 51
DOI 10.1007/978-1-4419-0090-6_4, © Springer Science+Business Media, LLC 2009

Why are Friends Needed?

Friends are important to girls' social and emotional well-being as they provide sources of activity, esteem, worth, and support. As confidantes, they provide emotional, social, and psychological support. Friends provide task or instrumental support when they lend each other money or clothes to wear and help each other to get her chores done. Cognitive support is provided when they offer opinions and advise on personal issues. Lastly, friends can provide an outlet for intimacy and a means in which to enhance interpersonal skills (Way, 1996).

Whether in person or utilizing technology (instant messaging, texting, etc.) communicating is a large part of the adolescent girl's social world. Popular sites such as FaceBook and MySpace can provide an infinite number of friends, and girls can avoid awkward social interactions through these mediums. Adolescent girls require more social time than boys, and friends provide this social outlet. This is especially apparent during early adolescence when belonging and fitting in is very important. Girls who are isolated and who do not have friends are more likely to have lower self-esteem and other interpersonal problems than those with friends (Pagano & Hirsch, 2007). The relational orientation of girls is one of the reasons why friendship is so critical during this period.

Friends Provide Needed Relationships

As discussed in Chapter 2, females are relational and derive their sense of self from relationships with others. Girls and women feel good (or bad) about themselves based in part on their relationships with significant others in their lives. Males, on the other hand, are not as dependent on these relationships to feel good about themselves, and subsequently, their need for social contact is not as great. Males in early adolescence tend to focus on activities more so than talking and relationships. Male friends are more likely to come together to play video games, sports, or like activities rather than to share secrets and intimacies as girls do when they come together.

During early adolescence, girls have a desire to spend more time with friends and peers and during this period, they begin to develop friendship bonds that may be long lasting. Rejection is usually inevitable as most girls are not always included by everyone. The next section discusses friendship patterns among African American girls, followed by discussions of romantic relationships, the negative side of relationships, and then an examination of peer influence on three categories of behavior, sexual activity, drug use, and academic achievement.

Friendship Patterns

Developmental Aspect of Friendships

Children, as young as 3 or 4 years old, show preferences for being with other children and use the word "friend." In fact, about 75% of preschoolers have friendships that are identified by their mothers or nursery school teachers (Hartup & Stevens, 1999). Across all developmental periods, friendships are important, but they are especially so during adolescence. Among teenagers, 80–90% report having mutual friends. This includes one or two best friends and several good friends (Hartup & Stevens, 1999). One of the reasons middle school may be difficult for girls is because this is the time that groups and cliques form, and girls strive to make sure they are in the "right" group. As they mature and transition from middle to high school, they gain a better perspective on themselves and rely less on their friendship and peer group for self-definition.

What do Same-Sex Friendship Networks Look Like?

During adolescence, girls tend to choose friends who are similar in values, interests, and extracurricular activities (Hamm, 2000). During this period, the formation of friendships is influenced by convenience, i.e., where the girls live and attend school. Girls spend more time with their friends during middle childhood and adolescence than during any other time period. During early and middle childhood, the number of best friends varies from three to five. During this time, girls tend to have a smaller number of friends and a more exclusive network than boys. This reverses in later adolescence as during later adolescence, girls have a larger network of good friends than boys. The number of friends remains fairly constant through adolescence and early adulthood (Hartup & Stevens, 1999).

For African Americans girls, ethnicity is one factor in friendship choice. African American girls tend to have friends of the same ethnic group even when they are in ethnically diverse environments. Factors that influence friendship choice among African American youth may differ than factors that influence friendship choice among girls in other ethnic groups. For example, African American youth may reject friendships from other African Americans whom they feel "act white." Acting white consists of behaviors that are not necessarily negative but may be considered desirable in the White community. Some of these behaviors include getting good grades, dressing in a certain way, and participating in certain extracurricular activities (Fordham & Ogbu, 1986). Socioeconomic factors (whether real or perceived) may affect how adolescents choose friends. While some African American girls reject friendship from those considered as "acting white," this rejection is more likely to occur among African American males than females. "Acting white" to African

American girls does not typically include getting good grades but refers to how a girl dresses, her hair style, and hanging out with "White friends."

Cliques

Cliques are one type of friendship. Dolcini and Adler (1994) examined adolescent cliques in an urban African American neighborhood. Cliques were defined as small, close-knit groups ranging in number from 3 to 10 with youth similar in age, gender, and race. One-hundred-thirteen friends were interviewed for this study. The authors found that about half of the youth were in cliques, and about one-fifth were in dyads only. The other adolescents did not associate with friends. The average clique comprised four youth of the same age and ethnicity, and they had relatively longstanding relationships. Cliques were characterized as having high trust levels, and girls within cliques supported each other instrumentally (e.g., with material things) as well as emotionally. Forming cliques allows girls to reject others and reaffirm their own positive identity like an exclusive country club.

Respect and Trust

A key component of a strong and mutually satisfying friendship is respect and trust. Unfortunately, many African American girls perceive (whether true or otherwise) that they cannot trust their peers and girl friends. The quote at the beginning of this chapter illustrates this.

Way (1996) conducted interviews with 24 urban youth (boys and girls). The majority were African American from poor or working-class families. Participants were interviewed at three time periods, once each in the ninth, tenth, and eleventh grades. The interview protocol included questions about friendship such as "Do you have close friends, and if so, what is this friendship like?" Way noted that almost all the interviewees, 21 out of 24, reported distrusting their same-sex peers. These adolescents mentioned difficulties of finding same-sex peers who would be there for them, who would keep their secrets, and who would not steal their romantic partners. Girls were more likely than boys to report that they had difficulty trusting same-sex peers, but they still maintained a close or best friendship with at least one other person of the same-sex. Way speculated that a violation of friendship was a factor in giving up on all friends for boys, but a violation of friendship among girls did not have such as effect. She speculated that this may be due to the way girls are socialized to have close friendships. Girls are willing to maintain and/or find new friendships even when they have experienced betrayals and violations of this friendship.

In my observations of girls involved in our intervention programs (and also in interviews), I have also noticed the theme of distrust of other girls. The girls we have talked to have reported that they cannot trust other girls to keep confidential information, often commenting on how other girls will put their "business" in the street. Perhaps it is because of the interpersonal and communal orientation of girls that violations of trust and respect are especially salient (Way). Because positive female relationships are important, components of our intervention program for African American girls have addressed this issue by focusing on how to be a good friend to other girls (discussed later).

Interracial Friendships

Most children and adolescents have a preference for friends from the same racial and ethnic group (Scott, 2004). However, interracial friendships exist although they are often dependent upon the context and where people live. Interracial friendships tend to occur when girls from different racial and ethnic groups live in the same community and attend the same school. While there are many benefits of interracial friendships, including exposure to other cultures and reduction in stereotyping (Ponterotto, Utsey, & Pedersen, 2006), there are also some challenges.

Scott (2004) discussed the potential challenges that can occur with friendships among African American and White girls. She noted that friendships between African American and White girls may cause some conflicts because of cultural differences in what each group considers socially important. According to Scott (2004), in White female-dominated peer groups, girls who are considered physically attractive, have relatively high family wealth, are considered smart, tend to have higher social status and more desirable friends than those who do not have these characteristics. These characteristics may not be as important to social status for African American girls because cultural norms and values may not dictate wealth and attractiveness as important attributes for success and status in the African American community. African American girls may value talent and creative ability more and find attractive attributes such as dressing well, being a good dancer as attractive. Thus, Scott noted that, equalitarian friendships between African American and White girls are challenging to nurture and sustain. In overview, positive interracial friendships can exist and generally are dictated by where the girls live and go to school. However, cultural differences in values might play a role in the quality and sustainability of these friendships.

Internet Friendships

With computers and internet accessible in most homes, the internet has become a popular medium for initiating and maintaining relationships. In 2006, 89% of teens accessed the internet from home. Ninety-three percent used the internet as a place for social interaction to share artistic creations, tell stories, and interact with others (Lenhart et al., 2007). MySpace, FaceBook, and other social networking internet sites are frequently used by teens to communicate with existing friends and to meet new ones. While these sites provide opportunities for teens with similar interest to network with each other, there have been some concerns with sexual predators, and safeguards should be put in place to guard against this. Information specific to social network sites for African American girls could not be identified, but it is likely that her networking patterns are similar to that of other teens.

Romantic Friendships

During early and middle adolescence, youth become increasingly interested in dating and romantic relationships. Generally, by the age of 14 or 15, most adolescents have had some experience with dating (Connolly & Johnson, 1996). A romantic relationship supports healthy psychosocial development and contributes to adjustment and well-being in many domains (Zimmer-Gembeck, Siebenbruner, & Collins, 2001). A romantic relationship can bring about increases in self-confidence, interpersonal skills, and communication. On the other hand, romantic relationships can have some negative outcomes when it leads to premature sexual activity and negative influences from male partners.

Dating Initiation

There are gender and ethnic differences in regard to the developmental timing of dating and romantic relationships. Although African American girls become sexually active at a younger age, they typically date at an older age than White girls. Regan and colleagues (2004) explored the timing of early romantic attachments such as first dates, falling in love, and sexual intercourse. The authors were interested in whether there were gender and ethnic differences in the onset and age at which these activities were first experienced. Six-hundred-eighty-three male and female college students completed questionnaires and indicated the age at which they had been on a date, had a serious romantic relationship, and had sexual intercourse. The authors found that African Americans were more likely to go on their first date at a later average age (17.53 years) than other ethnic groups. Whites were more likely to go on their first date at the youngest age (14.53 years), then Hispanics at 15.75 years, and Asians at 16.12 years. African American and White participants reported engaging in intercourse at about the same time (average age was 16.31 years for African Americans and 16.97 years for Whites). This age was lower than that for Latinos at 17.33 years and Asians at 18.85 years. This research illustrates the disconnect between dating and sexual activity among African American girls.

Romantic and dating relationships are often a prelude to sexual activity during adolescence (Miller & Moore, 1990). Adolescents who date on a more consistent basis have more opportunities and access to potential sexual partners, thereby increasing the likelihood that they will have sex (Davies & Windle, 2000; Longmoe, Manning, & Giordano, 2001). In fact, frequent dating at an early age is linked with younger sexual experience (Dorius, Heaton, & Steffen, 1993; Miller et al., 1997). Consequences of sexual experiences are discussed in more detail in Chapter 9.

Preference for Dating Partners

Smith (1996) explored characteristics of ideal dating partners of 81 urban African American high school students. Smith cited earlier research that had shown that African American students rated materialistic factors (e.g., money, education) more important than White students who rated personality traits more highly (Hansen, 1977). Additionally, earlier studies had found that males and females preferred different characteristics in dating partners (Goodwin, 1990). Smith examined students' ratings of perceived importance of 12 preselected characteristics. Students were asked to rate the importance of certain traits and characteristics that they might find in a potential dating partner. For example, students read the statement "I would like to date someone who is ..." (e.g., "honest," "athletic"). Then, students checked one of three responses: "Very Important," "Somewhat Important," or "Not Important" beside each phrase.

Smith found that overall students placed more importance on interpersonal qualities than materialistic qualities, such as having a nice car. This was true for both males and females. Both males and females ranked the traits of honesty and being caring highest in importance followed closely by "fun to talk to" and "sense of humor." The author noted that there were only slight differences in average rank orderings for males and females, with the exception that males were more likely to rate "good looking" higher than females.

The Smith study is somewhat outdated and more recent research is needed on this topic. In Chapter 9, on Sexuality and its Consequences, I review the study by Ashcraft (2004) in which African American girls reported that they expected material things (e.g., getting nails and hair done, clothes, entertainment, etc.) when in a relationship with a male. These findings suggest that young adolescent females might prefer materialistic attributes more so than personality characteristics. However, girls in the Ashcraft study resided in a low-income community, and perhaps materialistic things are desired more so when there are fewer resources in the home and community. Their models may have also modeled such preferences.

Dating and Academic Achievement

While there are some positive benefits derived from dating (e.g., increased self-esteem, intimacy needs met, opportunities for negotiation), there are also some negative outcomes associated with dating.

Quatman, Sampson, and Robinson (2001) examined the relationship between dating status and academic achievement among students in 8th, 10th, and 12th grades. The findings from this study indicated that adolescents who dated frequently (more than once or twice a month) had lower levels of academic achievement and academic motivation than adolescents who did not date frequently. This trend was consistent for boys and girls and relatively young (8th grade) or more mature (10th and 12th grades) students. Because the participants in this study were mostly White and Asians, we are uncertain if dating affects academic achievement among African American girls as it does for girls from other ethnic groups.

Interracial Dating

Although there are increases in interracial dating, overall, adolescents are similar to adults and prefer dating and marrying within their own racial and ethnic groups. While there have been more positive attitudes toward interracial dating and relationships, some stigma continues to exist within families and communities (Gaines, 2001). Mok (1999) reported that parental disapproval is often an obstacle in initiating and maintaining an interracial relationship. Wong, Kao, and Joyner (2006) predicted and found that adolescents in interracial relationships (compared to intraracial relationships) perceived less support from families, and consequently, the relationship was more likely to dissolve quicker.

Data from the National Longitudinal Study of Adolescent Health were used to examine relationship stability in interracial dating. The sample consisted of about 5,000 males and 5,000 females with a mean age of 16. About 24% of the sample was African American, 62% was White, 8% was Hispanic, 5% was Asian, and less than 1% was Native American. Wong and colleagues found that adolescents who dated interracially were more likely to keep the relationship to themselves; they were less likely to publicly show their attraction to each other; they were less likely to talk to their mother about their romantic partner; and they were less likely to meet their partner's parents than those in same racial group relationships. The authors conclude that interracial dating is still not accepted by families of these adolescents and society in general. However, many interracial relationships are maintained, and more research may be needed to understand how these relationships survive overtime.

The Negative Side of Peers and Friendships

Although having friends is generally beneficial, friends can also be costly. Friendships with mutually reciprocal individuals who are well adjusted are important sources of emotional and psychological support for adolescents. However, friendships with poorly adjusted individuals can be a drain on an adolescent's energy and resources. Poorly adjusted friends are also more likely than well-adjusted friends to engage in problem behaviors. And poorly adjusted friends may also create barriers to finding and maintaining relationships with more well-adjusted friends.

Friendship brings with it both closeness and conflicts. Mutual self-disclosure and social support found in adolescent friendships can foster the development of intimate and fulfilling relationships. On the other hand, conflict, inevitable in almost all friendships, can lead to betrayals and sometimes, emotional hurt (Pagano & Hirsch, 2007).

It is not uncommon for friends to be jealous of each other's achievements. Social comparison theory (Festinger, 1954) and the self-evaluation maintenance model (Tesser, 1988) predict that we will feel worse about the accomplishments of those who are similar to us than those who are not similar. When we compare ourselves to similar others who are better than us, it makes our own shortcomings salient. It is this social comparison that girls are sensitive to as we have often heard "she is jealous," "she does not like the fact that I have a boyfriend," etc.

Gangs

Gangs provide a means in which a girl's relationship and affiliation needs are met. Gangs provide safety and other instrumental needs such as money, entertainment, and protection. While historically gangs have consisted of males, they are attracting more females. According to a National Youth Gang Survey conducted in 2000, approximately 6% of the almost 773,000 documented active gang members were female. Other studies suggest that the percentage of female gang members range from 8% to 38%.

Peer pressure is one of the factors contributing to gang involvement among African American girls. Walker-Barnes and Mason (2001) explored gang involvement among ethnic minority females. Thirty-one ethnic minority girls who attended school in a high-crime urban community were interviewed and asked reasons why adolescents join gangs. The most commonly reported reason for female gang involvement was peer pressure. Interviewees also reported that girls joined gangs because they desired protection from neighborhood crime, because they came from dysfunctional families, and because they desired protection against other gangs. Girls from families with low family cohesion and high family conflict were more likely to join gangs than girls with high family cohesion and support. Also, gangs, through their participation in illegal activities, were seen as providing access to excitement and money-making opportunities not available in legitimate ways. Finally, adolescents may view gang membership as a way of obtaining respect.

Li, Stanton, & Pack (2002) further explore some of the risk and protective factors associated with gang involvement among urban African American adolescents. They collected data from 349 urban African American youth (age: 9–15 years). Differences in exposure to violence, resilience, and distress symptoms between gang members and nonmembers were examined. In addition, the researchers examined whether these distress symptoms were due to the risk behaviors or involvement in the gang itself. Youth with current or past gang membership had higher levels of risk involvement, lower levels of resilience, higher exposure to violence, and higher distress symptoms. The Li et al. study provides evidence that gang membership itself may be associated with increased risk and poor psychological functioning. Safe community environments and constructive after-school activities, including employment opportunities, are needed to reduce pressure to keep girls from gang involvement especially in high-risk communities.

Also, parents can play a large role in deterring their adolescent girl from gang involvement. In a longitudinal study, Walker-Barnes and colleagues examined whether peers or parents had the greatest influence on gang involvement. They also looked at how gang involvement changed over time and whether gang involvement differed across ethnic groups. They found that, in general, youth decreased their level of gang involvement over the course of the school year. Adolescent gang involvement and gang-related delinquency were most strongly related to peer gang involvement and peer gang delinquency. However, parenting behavior also contributed to gang involvement and delinquency, even after considering peer behavior. The effect of parenting was especially salient for African American parents. When parents had high levels of behavioral control of their adolescent and less lax control, their children were less likely to be involved in gangs and in gang delinquency. The study by Walker-Barnes and colleagues suggests that there are things parents can do to reduce delinquency and gang involvement even when residing in low-resource communities. African American parents can lessen the chances of their children becoming involved with gangs and delinquency if they know where their children are when they are not in school, know who their friends are, and enforce curfews. Parental monitoring and supervision of girls appear to be critical elements of keeping her out of a gang.

Birds of a Feather Flock Together

Adolescents with similar interests and goals tend to find one another and form peer groups around salient parts of their identity, sharing similar beliefs and attitudes (Fuligni, Eccles, Barber, & Clements, 2001). Peers tend to engage in similarly negative or positive behaviors. In general, youth with friends who smoke, drink, and use other drugs are more likely to engage in the same behaviors. However, while there are some similarities among friends, African American youth tend to be less similar to their friends than youth from other ethnic groups (Hamm, 2001; Tolson & Urberg, 1993). Moreover, African American girls (compared to girls from other ethnic/racial groups) may select friends based on different criteria. Peer and friend influence on drug use, sexual activity, and academic achievement is discussed next. Included in this discussion is some of the research conducted by my graduate students on the topic of peer influence.

Drug Use

While overall there is similarity among peers with regard to drug use, the influence of friends' drug use on African American adolescent drug use may be weaker than for Whites (Unger, 2001; Wallace & Muroff, 2002). Families may be more influential in smoking and the use of other drugs among African American youth relative to youth from other ethnic groups (Wallace & Muroff, 2002). For example, in one study, Dornelas and colleagues (2004) found that African American teens (50%) were more likely to smoke with family members than White (25%) or Latino (5%) teens. While peers and friends continue to influence smoking and other drug use, the research suggests that the degree of this influence may not be as great among African American youth as youth from other ethnic groups.

In a dissertation study, Boyd (2003) examined the direct and the indirect impacts of peer support and family support on drug and sex refusal efficacy among African American girls. The study recruited 155 African American sixth-grade girls residing in an urban community. Boyd found that parental support (from fathers) and not peer support was correlated with higher drug refusal efficacy. This finding supports the need for positive father–daughter relationships. Boyd also found that the quality of parental relationships with their daughter correlated with peer support. Girls who had positive parental relationships reported positive types of peer support. The results suggest that perhaps parents are guiding and/or structuring opportunities that encourage girls to interact with positive peers. However, girls in this study were relatively young (11–12 years), and this might not be the case with older adolescents.

In a recent study, Clark, Nguyen, and Belgrave (2008) examined the role of peer risk and protective factors along with individual, family, and community risk and protective factors for alcohol and marijuana use. They were specifically interested in determining whether peers might influence alcohol and marijuana use differently for those who lived in urban versus rural communities. The sample consisted of over 900 African American youth who participated in a state-wide assessment of risk and protective factors for drug use. The authors did not examine gender differences in this study. They found that peer risk and protective factors were more influential in alcohol and marijuana use among urban youth. On the other hand, family and community protective and risk factors were more related to alcohol and marijuana use among rural youth. Peers are very proximal to urban youth and thus may have more opportunities to exert influence than among rural youth.

The research by Clark and colleagues did not specifically look at African American girls, so we do not know if the degree of friend and peer influence is the same for girls as for boys. Clearly modeling by parents along with social pressure to use drugs among friends are two factors that should be considered in drug prevention effects.

Sexual Activity

Friends impact sexual behavior of adolescent girls through several mechanisms. Sharing intimate details is a way girls cement the band of friendship. Girls socialize each other as to what to expect from a dating relationship, what the norms might be regarding intimate encounters, and what to do to protect themselves against sexually transmitted infections (Harper et al., 2004) (also see Chapter 9).

Girls talk to their best friends about their dating and sexual relationships. Harper and colleagues (2004) interviewed 15 African American adolescent girls from a large West Coast City about their communication with their closest friends about dating and sexual activity. Girls reported that they were initially reluctant and embarrassed to tell their close friends about their sexual activity. But once a detail was shared, with coaxing, they would tell the whole story. Males, on the other hand, were more likely to speak openly and casually about their sexual activity without prompting from friends. They frequently bragged about their sexual conquests and the frequency of sexual activity.

Females and males tended to describe their dating and sexual activity in different ways. Females used relational terms in their description such as "they did it," and the words used to describe the experience captured the dyadic relationship between the couple. Males, on the other hand, tended to share information with their close friends regarding females whom the friends wanted to pursue for sex. Their discussion often focused on the likelihood that a particular female would agree to have sex with them. Terms used when talking about sexual activity were more self-based and involved the male receiving something such as "he got some" or doing something to the female. These types of comments suggested that in general males were less likely than females to report that the sexual activity was a mutual act.

Academic Achievement

Academic achievement is another area in which friends tend to be similar with some exceptions that will be noted. Across most racial and ethnic groups, friends tend to have similar levels of academic achievement. For example, students who associated with high-achieving peers in the Fall semester of an academic school year show increases in academic interest and improvements in achievement after 1 year of socializing with these high-achieving peers (Mounts & Steinberg, 1995). African American youth may be more likely to socialize with peers who are more engaged in out-of-school activities than classroom activities. Consequently, similar levels of academic achievement among friends may not be the norm. This may be partly due to the fact that in academic settings, African American students may not receive the type of affirmation and support that academic achievement brings for members of other ethnic groups (Steele, 1992). Furthermore African American students, especially males who choose to identify with academic success, are not always supported by their peers (Fordham & Ogbu, 1986; Ogbu, 1991). Among White youth, the most popular students tend to be those who are academically successful. Among African American youth, the most popular students are not those who are the most academically successful. Thus, African Americans youth may minimize the importance of school success and attend to other dimensions when selecting peers and friends (Graham, Taylor, and Hudley, 1998).

Hamm (2000) investigated academic similarity among African American, Asian American, and European American adolescents and their nominated (i.e., classmates they liked) friends. Similarity for academic orientations was moderate but significantly greater for European American and Asian American adolescents than for African American adolescents and their nominated friends, for whom academic similarity was significant but low. The author speculated that the lower similarity between African American adolescents and their nominated friends on academic orientations is consistent with earlier research that have shown that this dimension is not as important for African American adolescents.

However, having friends who engage in risky behavior may be a risk factor for poor academic achievement among African American youth. Stanard, Belgrave, and Corneille (2008) studied 184 African American adolescent females and 127 males living in an urban community. Stanard and colleagues were interested in whether peer risky behavior affected academic orientation, interests, and grades of students. The authors found that students who had peers engaged in risky behavior (e.g., being suspended from school, using drugs, being sexually active, drinking) had lower school engagement themselves. Youth who had peers and friends engaged in risky behavior were less likely to report high levels of academic interests and achievement. In summary, girls tend to chose friends who are similar in values, interests, and lifestyles. Girls also chose friends who display similar risky behaviors, including drug use and sexual activity. However, African American girls may be less likely than girls from other ethnic groups to choose friends based on academic similarity.

Promoting Positive Relationships Among Girls

As discussed, relationships are central to all females. Relationships may be especially critical to the social and psychological well-being of African American females because of relational values and Africentric values of communalism and interdependence (Belgrave & Allison, 2006). Therefore, a major component of our intervention programming with African America girls has been to increase positive relationships among girls. The Sisters of Nia curriculum was developed to increase positive relationships among girls and supportive female adults (Belgrave, Cherry, Botler & Townsend, 2008). It can be used with girls who are aged 11–14. This curriculum, discussed in Chapter 2, also targets increased ethnic identity and androgynous gender roles. The 14 session curriculum has two sessions devoted specifically to relationship building among girls. The objective of the first session on relationship is (1) to help girls to begin to develop more positive relationships with other girls; (2) to increase cohesion, teamwork, and trust among girls; and

(3) to decrease any negative attitudes and behaviors girls might have toward each other. An additional two sessions titled "Mirror, Mirror, what are you a reflection of" provide an opportunity for girls to examine why they put down and say negative things about each other. Two of the proverbs we used to illustrate the importance of positive relationships are "show me your friend and I will show you your character" and "a sister is like a shoulder to cry on."

The process of implementing the program focuses on building positive relations among girls working together in small groups (approximately ten girls) to complete interdependent activities. Young African American adult females serve as facilitators and model to the girls how to cooperatively work together. Girls are rewarded based on the success of the group and are praised when they practice being a good sister to one another. One of the homework assignments asks the girls to practice being a sister friend to another girl who is not in the program. An evaluation of the program showed that girls decreased in relational aggression (verbally saying mean things, social exclusion) after participating in the program (Belgrave, Reed, & Plybon, 2004). In after-school programs that have used this curriculum, teachers and other school staff report that they have observed changes in how the girls related to each other within the school environment, both within the classroom and on the playground. That is, girls became more likely to help a girl out who had problems, to refrain from gossiping and talking about other girls, and to generally looking out for other girls (Cherry & Belgrave, 1999). More information about the Sisters of Nia Curriculum is in the "Resource" section.

Summary

Girls spend a considerable amount of time with friends and in peer groups. Friends are important to girls' social and emotional well-being. Friends provide needed relationships, self-worth, support, and activity partners. Adolescent girls need more social time than boys and friends provide this social outlet. Girls tend to choose friends who are similar in values, interests, and extracurricular activities. African American girls are less likely to choose friends who are similar academically and may choose friendships based on nonacademic interests and activities.

Respect and trust are important components of friendships for African American girls. There is limited research on this topic but the limited work suggests that feelings of distrust regarding peers exist among some African American girls.

Girls tend to be friends with girls from their own ethnic groups. There are positive aspects of interracial friendships but sometimes challenges when values differ.

In terms of romantic relationships, African American girls tend to go on their first date at an age older than girls in other ethnic groups. However, age of first sexual intercourse is similar to that for White girls. The literature is mixed with regard to whether African American girls prefer partners with positive personality attributes or partners who have more materialistic attributes. African American girls are more likely to date within their own ethnic/racial group, and although there have been some changes in attitudes toward interracial dating, some stigma still exists. In general, youth with friends who smoke, drink, and use other drugs are more likely to do so themselves. However, while there are some similarities among friends, African American youth, both males and females, tend to be less similar to their friends than youth from other ethnic groups. Among African American adolescents, peers may not be as influential as parents with regard to problem behaviors such as drug use. A program that has been used to increase positive relationships among girls is called "Sisters of Nia."

In conclusion, friends and peers are a strong link to African American girl's competency and achievement. Positive, prosocial, and mutually fulfilling friendships can support her psychosocial development, expectations, and well-being.

Recommendations and Resources

Increasing Positive Friendships Through Activities

Organized Sports and Athletics

Participating in organized sports and athletic activities are good ways for girls to make friends as these types of activities allow girls to share similar goals and activities. Additionally, girl athletes are much less likely to engage in problem behaviors, such as drug use and early sexual activity, when compared to girls who do not participate in sport and athletic activities.

Increasing Positive Relationships and Prosocial Behavior

Girl Scouts and Other Girl/Female Groups

These groups provide opportunities for girls to work together to promote civic and community responsibility. Most of these groups are involved in doing volunteer work within the community. This is a good way for teens to meet people outside their immediate friendship group and to learn how to support and be supported by others.

Preventing Gang Membership

There are several things parents can do to prevent gang involvement. Some of these include reporting suspicious activities to the police, sharing information with other parents, and ensuring that their daughters are involved in supervised, positive after-school and weekend activities. Also, family conflict and poor family communication may contribute to girls wanting to belong to gangs. See websites under "Resource" section for additional information on preventing gang involvement.

Interventions for Enhancing Positive Relationships

A few interventions have been developed and evaluated with regard to increasing positive friendships and peer relations for girls in early adolescence.

Sisters of Nia

This curriculum was developed by the author and colleagues based on the assumption that positive and fulfilling interpersonal relationships can serve as protective attributes for African American girls. The 14 sessions are designed to increase positive relationships among girls and the program facilitators. The Sisters of Nia Curriculum was described earlier in the text and can be obtained from Research Press (800 519–2707). www.researchpress.com

The Girls Circle is a structured support group for girls 9–18 years of age. The Girls Circle provides girls the opportunities to talk and to increase positive relationships with one another in a safe setting in which they can develop positive interpersonal relationships. The groups are generally held weekly for about 2 hours. A trained facilitator leads the group using a format that includes each girl taking turns and listening to each other talk about their concerns and interests. Girls further express their creativity through activities such as role playing, journaling, poetry, dance, etc. The program can be used in schools, religious institutions, after-school programs, community centers, homes, boys and girls clubs, etc. Further information on trainings can be obtained by viewing http://www.girlscircle.com/Traininglist.aspx and/or by contacting Girls Circle Association 707 794–9477.

Girls Inc. Friendly PEERsuasion® (GIFP) is an interactive prevention program aimed at helping girls in middle school (ages: 11–14) acquire knowledge, skills, and support systems to avoid substance abuse. While the program is targeted toward preventing substance abuse, it also increases girls' capacity to engage in positive relationships and to refrain from negative peer pressure. The program uses peer reinforcement and adult leadership to teach girls to respond critically to messages that encourage drug use. Girls participate in 14 one-hour-long curriculum sessions. More information can be obtained by contacting Linday Briggs, at Girls Incorporated, E-mail: lbriggs@girls-inc.org; Web site: http://www.girls-inc.org

Resources

The most recent gang-related resources may be found on the Office of Juvenile Justice and Delinquency Prevention's website (http://www.ojp.usdoj.gov/ojjdp or http://www.ojjdp.ncjrs.gov/)
by searching using the keyword "gang." Also, see the Office of Juvenile Justice and Delinquency Prevention Girls Study Group for information on prevention girl gang membership at
http://www.ncjrs.gov/pdffiles1/ojjdp/218905.pdf

Zimmerman, J., & Reavill, G. (1998). *Raising Our Athletic Daughters: How Sports Can Build
Self-Esteem and Save Girls' Lives.* New York: Mainstreet Books.

Chapter 5
Communities and Neighborhoods

One of the positives is that we do have police around here when we need them, even though they don't come around here, but that's their job is to be around. But one of the negatives is, it shouldn't be as many. Even though you need them, it shouldn't be that many. Because it should be like the crime shouldn't be so high, that's a negative. The crime shouldn't be so high that were we have to have police stationed like every five blocks, right around the corner from each other. But it seems like the world is getting more negative each day....

Teen focus Group Participant in Response to question, "what positive things happen in your community?"

The communities and neighborhoods girls reside in have a great impact on their beliefs, values, and actions. Community influence on African American adolescent girls is the focus of this chapter. A large part of any community is neighborhood schools and teachers, and these topics are also touched upon in this chapter. This chapter begins with definitions of neighborhood and community, discusses the role of poverty, then the influence of neighborhoods on academic achievement and expectations, drug use and violence, and sexual behavior. Community types differentially influence behaviors, and both urban and rural communities are discussed. Much research on African American youth living in urban communities has discussed the negative consequences of living in urban communities. Some of this research is discussed, and along with it, we include a discussion of community resources and assets. Rural communities present unique challenges and strengths, and they are also discussed. The chapter concludes with a summary followed by a recommendation and resource section.

The terms "neighborhood" and "community" are sometimes used interchangeably. Neighborhoods are defined both geographically and socially (Chaskin, 1998). A geographical definition of neighborhood can include proximity and localized settings within a community, within a larger city, town, or suburb as a basis for a neighborhood; it can also define neighborhood as a residential district (Wikipedia, 2008). Neighborhoods can also be defined as social communities with considerable face-to-face interaction among members. Characteristics of a neighborhood include geographical boundaries and also structural aspects that have to do with what the people in a neighborhood look like. These include characteristics such as the average education level, occupation, and income of residents. Other attributes include the percentage of home ownership, single-parent households, birth to teen mothers, poverty level, crime, and drugs. Neighborhoods can also be characterized functionally in terms of assets and interactions people have with one another. Examples of neighborhood attributes include how residents feel about each other, availability of medical and social services, neighborhood cohesion (e.g., degree of attachment to people and institutions in the community), and availability of after-school clubs and activities. Structural and functional neighborhood attributes will be discussed in relation to African American girls.

Community can be defined as a group of people with diverse characteristics who are linked by social ties, share common perspectives, and engage in joint action in geographical locations or settings (MacQueen et al., 2001). Community is also defined as a network of association of people, families, institutions, and organizations. Community as such is not just a geographical location but may be feelings that members have of belonging among people who share common interests such as the "African American community." The terms "community" and "neighborhood" are used interchangeably, and in this chapter, terms will be used to coincide with literature cited.

Understanding the Role of Poverty in Disadvantaged Communities

We begin with a discussion of poor and disadvantaged communities. The majority of the research on African American adolescents has been conducted with youth who reside in low-resource communities. In the psychological and social science literature on neighborhood and community, there is a widespread assumption that communities occupied by a majority of African American are "disadvantaged" communities and that youth residing in these communities generally end up with some type of problem behavior. This is not true and there is much variability in African American communities and among the people who reside within.

Poverty is perhaps the biggest attribute found in disadvantaged neighborhoods. Poverty is associated with lack of adequate housing, crime, drug use, unemployment, homelessness, abandoned buildings, and many other negative attributes within communities. Poverty is not the sole cause of negative outcomes but likely interact with other social conditions prevalent in poor communities to contribute to poor children's outcomes. These factors can include family problems such as family conflict, lack of monitoring and supervision, as well as school problems such as few resources and inadequate teacher training (Upchurch, Aneshensel, Sucoff, & Levy-Storms 1999).

An example of the impact of poverty on social problems, including youth drug use, was examined in a study by Duncan, Duncan, and Strycker (2002). These authors examined how social conditions such as poverty, number of stores selling alcohol, and neighborhood cohesion interacted in such a way that it contributed to drug use among African American and White youth from 55 neighborhoods. The authors found that higher poverty neighborhoods had more stores that sold alcohol and less social cohesion. Lower social cohesion was linked to the perception that there were more problems with youth alcohol and drug use. This perception in turn was positively related to youth drug-and-alcohol arrests. Drug-and-alcohol arrests are in part due to greater police presence in poor neighborhoods. This study demonstrates that it is not just one neighborhood factor that contributes to problem behaviors among youth but that, oftentimes, a complex set of factors interact with one another to produce problem behaviors. Poverty seems to be a critical ingredient found in neighborhoods in which there are youth problem behaviors.

In overview, one key attribute of most disadvantaged neighborhoods is poverty and its associated consequences. There are several influences that neighborhoods have on the behavior and functioning of girls, and these are discussed next.

Neighborhood Influences on Behaviors

There have been several studies of African American adolescent outcomes and levels of functioning in urban, inner city, and disadvantaged neighborhoods. Although urban does not necessarily mean inner city or disadvantaged, many studies have used these terms interchangeably. These studies generally point to lower levels of functioning for youth in urban or inner-city neighborhoods. This is certainly not always true and adolescent functioning even in the most disadvantaged neighborhood is not always negative. Community assets and resources along with personal and family assets and resources can buffer youth who live in disadvantaged neighborhoods. Some of these will be discussed in the recommendations and resources section. African American girls seem to experience the impact of disadvantaged neighborhoods differently than African American boys especially with regard to academic achievement which is discussed next.

Neighborhood Influences on Academic Achievement and Expectations

Neighborhood factors are linked to youth expectations and these, in turn, influence life-course expectations and achievement outcomes. Academic achievement and life-course expectations are discussed in more detail in Chapter 7.

Attributes of a neighborhood such as income level, education level, and single-parent household parenting status affect the academic expectations and achievement of African American girls. African American adolescents who live in low-income neighborhoods report lower educational aspirations and expectations than those living in more affluent neighborhoods (Ceballo et al., 2004). Adolescents who live in neighborhoods with more middle-class residents are more likely to believe that education is important than those who live in communities with neighborhoods of lower socioeconomic status. Girls who believe education is important exert greater academic effort than those who do not believe education is important (Ceballo et al., 2004).

The connection between the income and education of neighborhood residents and youth achievement and expectations can be explained in part by socialization. Adults in neighborhoods socialize children through role modeling. Girls growing up in neighborhoods in which there are highly educated women come to see education as normative. Girls who live in neighborhoods with women who are not educated are not exposed to these possibilities. Research has shown that neighborhood cohesion contributes to academic achievement among girls. Plybon and colleagues (2003) conducted a study that enrolled 84 African American girls (ages from 11 to 14) to determine how their perception of neighborhood cohesion was linked to academic achievement. They found that perception of neighborhood cohesion as measured by items such as "overall, I like my neighborhood very much" was associated with better grades and better perception of academic efficacy.

Some researchers have speculated that differences among African American males and females in academic and other expectations may be attributed to the different effects of the neighborhoods in which they live. As will be discussed in Chapter 6, African American females tend to have higher academic expectations and achievement than African American males. Mello & Swanson (2007) addressed the question of how adolescent expectations relate to perception of neighborhood quality, and how this relationship differed for males and females. The study involved approximately 3,000 low-income African American adolescents who provided information about their future educational and occupational expectations and perceptions of neighborhood quality. Neighborhood quality was assessed by asking participants whether incidents such as vandalism, unemployment, and drug use were problems in their neighborhood. Educational expectation was measured by the likelihood that participants expected to attain a high school diploma, a college degree, or a good job in 10 years. The authors found that higher expectations regarding educational and occupational achievement were correlated with a higher perception of neighborhood quality. The findings also suggested that for males more so than females, perception of poor neighborhood quality was linked to lower expectations regarding educational attainment. The more negative that males reported their neighborhood quality to be, the less likely they were to believe they would graduate from high school or go to college. African American girls may see a lot more positive role models in their communities (i.e., teachers, mothers) and males may see fewer positive male role models.

This study by Mello and Swanson is an important one as it suggested that African American adolescent females' expectations about their future educational possibilities are not as affected by the quality of the neighborhood as are African American males. Although girls appear to be more resilient than boys, there are still some adverse effects of poor neighborhoods on educational expectations for girls. In overview, African American adolescent girls' and boys' expectations are lowered as a result of living in disadvantaged neighborhoods. However, this disadvantage is less for girls than for boys. This may partially explain why academic expectation and achievement differ for African American girls and boys.

Neighborhood Influences on Drug Use and Violence

A fair amount of research has investigated how neighborhood factors affect alcohol and drug use among African Americans. In general, these studies show that the context of the neighborhood is a predictor of drug use among youth (Gruenewald, Millar, Ponicki, & Brinkley, 2000). Neighborhood risk factors, such as neighborhood disorganization, low neighborhood attachment, high rates of residential mobility, high rates of crime, and high population density, contribute to adolescent drug use (Jensen, 2004; Lambert et al., 2004). On the other hand, factors such as neighborhood cohesion, intergenerational networks, and community resources protect youth from drug use (Plybon et al., 2003).

Although African American youth do not consume more drugs than White youth, drugs are more available in predominately African American neighborhoods than in White neighborhoods. African Americans youth are more likely (1) to report that illicit drugs are easy to obtain; (2) to have seen someone selling drugs in their community; and (3) to have seen someone who was drunk or high (Wallace & Muroff, 2002). Legal substances are advertised and marketed to African Americans more so than to Whites through neighborhood advertisements, and store merchants are more likely to sell tobacco to minors in African American than White neighborhoods (Wallace, 1998). One study found greater availability of cigarettes in predominantly African American neighborhoods (Reid, Peterson, Lowe, & Hughey, 2005).

Drug use in poor communities has also been studied among African American girls. The findings from these studies are consistent with other findings that show drugs are more likely to be used when communities have objective indicators of risk (i.e., crime and unemployment) and also youth perceptions of risk. Girls in neighborhoods of high risk tend to approve of drugs more, have attitudes more tolerant of drug use, and to use drugs more. Those in neighborhoods with lower neighborhood risk tend to have more negative attitudes toward drug use and to also have higher efficacy for refusing drugs (Corneille & Belgrave, 2007). In disadvantaged neighborhoods, drug use may be normative and there may be easy access to drugs. As will be discussed later, factors such as parental support and ethnic identity may attenuate the effects of neighborhood risk on drug use.

Lambert and colleagues (2004) studied the association between perceived neighborhood disorganization (violence/safety and drug activity in neighborhood) and later substance use of students. The study surveyed students in seventh grade and then 2 years later when they were in ninth grade. The youth's perceptions of neighborhood disorganization in grade seven were linked to increased tobacco, alcohol, and marijuana use in grade nine. For females, this association was also mediated by their attitudes about drug use and perceptions of drug harmfulness. Greater perceived risk of drug use and disapproval of drug use were associated with less drug use. Girls who lived in high-risk neighborhoods and who believed that drugs were harmful and/or had negative attitudes toward drugs were less likely to use drugs. These findings suggest that both neighborhood factors and girls' beliefs about drugs affect drug using behavior. The implication of the findings from this study is that beliefs about drug use can be modified through education.

Girls who are at risk for problem behaviors because of other factors may be even more susceptible to the adverse influence of living in disadvantaged neighborhoods. In a study of timing of puberty and neighborhood disadvantage among girls in minority neighborhoods, Obeidallah et al. (2004) examined how early puberty, a risk factor for problem behaviors, interacted with neighborhood disadvantage to explain violence. Girls in this study were between the ages of 13 and 15. Neighborhood context consisted of a combination of factors such as percentage below poverty line, unemployment, on public assistance, etc. Puberty timing was measured by when girls had achieved menarche.

The findings of the Obeidallah et al. study indicated that adverse effects of early onset of puberty only occurred among girls who lived in neighborhoods of disadvantage. The authors wrote: "biological changes do not exist in isolation from the social context; girls who experienced two stresses (i.e., early maturation in neighborhoods of disadvantage) were at greatest risk of acting violently" (page 1465). This disadvantage remained even after considering other neighborhood and family attributes. Early maturing girls in disadvantaged neighborhoods may be subject to attention and negative peer pressure by older males, who may be delinquent. Also, disadvantaged neighborhoods may present more opportunities to engage in problem behaviors such as drug use, sexual activity, and delinquency.

In general, when other risk factors exist, including factors such as poor family functioning, poor and disadvantaged neighborhoods may be especially deleterious to African American girls' well-being.

Neighborhood Influences on Sexual Behavior

Neighborhood factors also influences sexual behavior. Girls who live in disadvantaged neighborhoods may have different markers for growing up and sexual initiation may occur earlier for these girls. Cooper and Guthrie (2007) examined sexual behaviors along with other health behaviors in a sample of 137 African American adolescents whose ages ranged from 12 to 18. Participants reported thoughts and feelings about their neighborhood, including perceptions of how tough their neighborhood was. Participants also reported if they had a mentor such as a teacher or minister within their neighborhood. The authors found that the perception of neighborhood toughness was related to more risky sexual behaviors, substance use, and more problem behaviors. However, having a mentor from the community was linked to less drug use and fewer problem behaviors. Cooper and Guthrie noted that having strong family ties, including monitoring, reduces the risk of living in a distressed neighborhood.

Neighborhood Influences on Other Outcomes

Neighborhood context is also a factor in how well youth do in other domains. Studies have shown that perceived neighborhood disorder is linked to mental health problems such as lower self-esteem (Haney, 2007). Health problems such as asthma and a higher incidence of sexually transmitted diseases have also been shown to occur more in poor neighborhoods even while controlling for other factors that might contribute to poor health (Cohen & Dawson, 1993). Undoubtedly poor family and community resources interact to affect these adverse outcomes. Community context also affects the level of physical activity girls engage in. Sports and recreational facilitates are often not as prevalent in distressed urban communities, and youth in these communities may spend more time indoors engaging in nonphysical activities such as watching television (Romero, 2005). Also as mentioned earlier, African American girls may not be able to participate in after-school activities because of sibling child care and other family responsibilities.

Community Resources and Assets

Neighborhoods can also contribute to positive youth development and well-being. Community resources and assets contribute directly and indirectly to the well-being of adolescents who live in disadvantaged communities. Kegler et al. (2005) identified several community assets associated with positive youth outcomes: (1) nonparental adult role models, (2) positive peer role models, (3) participation in groups/sports, (4) religious activity, and (5) community involvement. Studies have shown that positive adults in the community, involvement in religious and community activities, and positive peers are associated with less drug use, less sexual behavior, and less violence and delinquency (Kegler et al., 2005). And as discussed next, being involved in community activities is also linked to other positive outcomes for African American girls.

Involvement in Community Activities

Participating in community and after-school activities has positive benefits for most youth, including African American girls. Crosby et al. (2002) studied African American girls' participation in Black organizations and how this participation was linked to sexually protective behaviors such as having fewer partners and more sexual communication. Girls who participated in this study were sexually active, unmarried, and between the ages of 14 and 18. Girls were asked whether they were active in Black organizations or social groups. Fifty-five percent of the girls indicated that they were active in Black organizations. Girls who were active in Black organizations had a lower likelihood of engaging in sex with casual partners, lower likelihood of inconsistent contraceptive use with steady partners, and infrequent sexual activity. Girls who were not involved in community activities had more sexual partners and other risky sexual practices.

There are many reasons for the link between participation in community activities and lower sexual risk (Crosby et al., 2002). Girls who participate in community activities are likely to be more supervised and structured in their free time. Girls who are involved in Black organizations may also have higher levels of ethnic identity and feelings of belongingness. Ethnic identity is linked to less sexual risk (see Chapter 2). Also, girls who are active in Black organizations and social clubs may live in communities where more resources are available. Finally, girls who are involved in community activities may see and interact with positive adult role models.

Community-Based Prevention Programs

Community-based prevention programs may be especially helpful in preventing problem behaviors. These programs are likely to be most effective when they are developed with the collaboration of community members. An example of this type of program is one that targeted HIV prevention among African American adolescents. The project called Project Bridge, which stands for Bold, Ready, Intelligent, Dedicated, Guided, and Equipped, targeted middle school adolescents. This interesting community–university collaboration (Marcus et al., 2004) used community based participatory research to design and carry out a faith-based HIV/AIDS prevention program for African American adolescents. The first phase of this program involved a formation of a coalition involving youth from one church. The coalition later expanded to include the greater metropolitan community. The community including students, parents, and teachers was involved in providing critiques of the proposed project prior to the project being implemented. Components of the intervention included a life skills' training components, a sex education component, a skill development component, and a peer component whereby youth had opportunities to organize and lead activities themselves.

The results of the BRIDGE program showed significant gains for several individuals who were involved in the process. The church community benefited from additional resources that could facilitate the training of youth (e.g., audiovisual equipment); staff at the church also developed the capacity to deliver HIV prevention and skill development training; and the program continued after grant funding was over. The youth at the church participated in the process of grant development and management of federal funds and increased their capacity to recognize good programs and assess their values. Students who participated in the intervention increased in their HIV knowledge and communication and decreased in their drug use. The university faculty benefited also from being trained in learning skills in negotiating and collaborating with community-based organizations. This program is a good example of a community-based prevention effort that had a positive effect across many community levels and types of persons. This program like many was implemented within an urban setting. Urban communities are discussed next.

Urban Communities

The vast majority of research has been conducted on youth who reside in urban communities. Urban communities are defined as all territory, population, and housing units located within an urbanized area or urban cluster (U.S. Census Bureau, 2000). An urbanized area and urban cluster include "core census block groups or blocks that have a population density of at least 1,000 people per square mile and surrounding census blocks that have an overall density of at least 500 people per square mile (U.S. Census Bureau, 2000). As discussed next, there are some unique challenges girls who live in urban communities face. Stress is one of these.

Stress in Urban Context

Youth in different communities experience different types of stress. For example, youth in an inner city may confront stressors of an unsafe neighborhood, juggling bus and train schedules, and changing neighbors due to more residential mobility. Youth in rural communities may have stressors of few employment opportunities, the lack of accessible transportation, and limited recreational activities and facilities (Allison et al., 1999).

It appears that stress is greater for African American youth than for White youth who live in urban areas. In an earlier study, Garrison, Schoenback, Shuulchter and Kaplan (1987), surveyed 735 African American and White adolescents between the ages of 11 and 17 living in an urban area. African American adolescents reported more negative life events than White adolescents. These included the death, divorce, or separation of a parent, death of a sibling, grandparent, or close friend, hospitalization of self or sibling, birth of a sibling, parental job loss, school failure and suspension, moving to a new school, juvenile court involvement, etc.

Brown, Powell, and Earls (1989) studied the ways in which community stress is linked to mental health symptoms among African American girls. Data were gathered from a survey administered to 1,347 African American female adolescents who lived in urban communities. The survey obtained information on nine major life stress events experienced over the previous 12 months. The events included serious threats to friends or relatives, serious financial problems, illness, handicap, legal problems, death, and injury. The findings revealed significant correlations among stress levels and mental and social well-being. Higher levels of stress were linked to more depression and acting out behavior.

Stress affects the body physiologically as well as psychologically. Kliewer, Wilson, and Plybon (2002) examined the relationship between neighborhood quality and increased blood pressure in response to stress among 77 African American adolescents with a mean age of 14. In this experiment, African American adolescents were subjected to a stressful task (a cold-face stimulus task) to determine blood pressure reactivity scores. The authors found poorer neighborhood quality was linked to increases in both systolic and diastolic blood pressure for females and decreases in blood pressure for males following the stressor. These findings suggested that African American girls may have a stronger physiological reaction to stress than boys. Perhaps boys who live in urban environments have become more attenuated to stressors and therefore show less reactivity.

In overview, living in an urban environment can be stressful for girls. On the other hand, there are several factors that might modulate how the adolescent experiences and copes with stress. These factors are discussed next.

Coping with Stress in Disadvantaged Neighborhoods

Disadvantaged community settings do not always result in unfavorable adolescent outcomes such as violence and drug use. Many parents and adolescents find ways to cope with adversities, including the potential violence of living in low-resource communities. In one study, Howard and colleagues (2003) talked to mostly African American parents of adolescent children who resided in a public housing development. The sample included 38 parents whose children ranged in ages from 10 to 16. These parents were asked to appraise potential violence in their community. The authors report that parents understood and were aware of the potential dangers in the neighborhood such as drug trafficking and gun violence. They found that parent and child communication was one way in which parents were able to learn about their children's exposure to violence. Parents also observed changes in their children's behaviors and activities such as not wanting to go outside, and wanting to stay with family members who did not live in the neighborhood. Parents used a variety of coping mechanics to cope with the stressors of community violence. They talked to their child about the dangers of the neighborhood and where to go and who to stay away from. They also communicated tough love letting the child know if she/he got in trouble they would not come to their rescue. Parents also monitored their children's behavior. They enforced curfews and knew who their child was with at all times. Sometimes parents became involved in helping to resolve their child's conflict. This included parental message that fighting was not always in their best interest, talking to the other child's parents, and sometimes involving the police and the housing authorities. Parents also used community resources for support. Some parents enrolled their children in community enrichment and recreational programs, clubs, and the like. In summary, it appears that parents use a variety of coping methods to help their children deal with stressors of living in low-resource communities.

Exposure to Community Violence

Most of the research on violence exposure and witnessing violence has been conducted on youth who reside in urban neighborhoods. Exposure to community violence is a stressor, and this exposure is associated with a range of problems. Exposure to violence in the community leads to several adverse outcomes such as anxiety, depression, symptoms of posttraumatic disorder, lower academic achievement, and drug use (Kliewer, 2006). Research by Kliewer (2006) shows that exposure to community violence has a physiological cost as well. Moreover, the effects of this exposure may differ for African American girls and boys.

Being victimized or witnessing violence is stressful. Therefore, Kliewer was interested in the relation between exposure to community violence and cortisol levels among African American youth. When stressed, cortisol is released as it supports the increase in attention and energy needed to cope. One-hundred-one African American youth with a mean age of 11 comprised the sample. The majority of the participants in her study resided in public housing communities within moderate-to high-violence areas within a southeastern City. Cortisol level was collected via a saliva sample. Other measures were collected including violence exposure (e.g., whether the participant had witnessed violence), major life stressors, and anxiety and depression. Parents, mostly mothers, were also surveyed about their child's behavior.

Kliewer found that the level of violence exposure was correlated with cortisol responses and that this varied as a function of gender. Specifically, she found that witnessing violence was associated with a cortisol-awakening response in girls but not boys. This may be due to the fact that boys are socialized to be tough and thus may be more desensitized to violence. This finding is supported by another study in which adolescent girls who were exposed to community violence had more anxiety symptoms such as difficulty in concentrating than boys (White et al., 1998).

In general, girls in high-risk communities are exposed to violence less frequently than boys. In spite of lower exposure, girls are more likely than boys to experience stress and other symptoms such as anxiety and depression when they are exposed to community violence (Foster, Kuperminc, & Price, 2004). There are different types of stressor and risk and protective factors for youth who reside in rural communities and this is discussed next.

Rural Communities

Rural communities are defined as communities that are located outside urbanized areas and clusters (USDA, 2004). There has been less written on African American rural youth, especially females. In spite of the fact that most studies have been published on urban African American youth and girls, rural youth also face many challenges. Some of these challenges are linked to poorer socioeconomic conditions in rural communities such as fewer resources and after-school activities. There also may be less entertainment and recreational activities, including fewer movie theatres, malls, teen clubs, and other places for rural youth to hang out.

Rural youth have different types of community experiences and different risk factors and assets may influence whether they engage in problem behaviors. A few studies have examined risk and protective factors among rural African American youth in regard to substance use and risky sexual behavior. For example, Nasim, Belgrave, Corona, & Townsend (2008) found that family factors were more influential in predicting substance use for rural rather than urban youth, while neighborhood risk factors were more predictive of substance use among urban youth.

In a recent study, Clark, Nguyen, and Belgrave (2008) examined risk and protective factors for alcohol and marijuana use among African American rural and urban youth. They were interested in whether neighborhood and other factors had different or the same influence on alcohol and marijuana use among urban and rural adolescents. Clark and colleagues examined individual, peer, family, and neighborhood risk and protective factors for alcohol and marijuana use among 10th and 12th graders who lived in urban and rural communities. They found that family and community risk/protective factors were associated with alcohol and marijuana use among rural youth. Peer and individual risk/protective factors were more likely (than community and family) to be linked to drug use among urban youth.

One of the reasons why community protective factors may be associated with less drug use is because there is less residential mobility in rural communities. Although people living in rural communities may be more geographically dispersed, there may be frequent contact with neighbors, and reliance on neighbors for looking out for one another. In rural communities there is also less mobility and neighbors may establish long-term relationships, interact more, and provide support to each other (Coleman, Ganong, Clark, & Madsen, 1989). Neighbors in rural communities may monitor the children in these communities since they know them well. These patterns led to strong community ties and supportive adults in rural more so than urban communities.

Research on drug use among youth from rural and urban communities shows mixed findings with some studies suggesting greater drug use among rural youth and other studies citing more drug use among urban youth. The national household and drug survey reports similar rates of cigarettes and alcohol among rural and urban youth but slightly higher rates of alcohol use among urban youth (SAMHSA, 2005). One area in which African American girls from rural communities tend not to fare as well as girls from urban communities is in the area of early and risky sexual activity. This is discussed next.

Rural Communities and Risky Sexual Behavior

As discussed in Chapter 9, African American teen females have higher rates of sexual initiation and sexual activity than teens in other ethnic groups. Moreover, there are differences in rural and urban communities in regard to early and risk sexual behavior. Milhausen and colleagues (2003) examined rural and nonrural African American high school students' sexual-risky behaviors using national data collected from the 1999 Youth Risk Survey. The sample consisted of 2,083 African American female high school students (359 from rural and 1,724 from nonrural communities). The sample also included African American males (304 from rural and 1,589 from nonrural communities). The study found significant differences between sexual behavior of rural and nonrural African American adolescent females. Rural African American females reported higher levels of risky behavior than urban African American females along several dimensions. For example, rural female adolescents were 46% more likely than urban females to report ever having sexual intercourse. Approximately 74.1% of rural females reported having sexual intercourse as compared to 60.7% of nonrural females. Rural females were 44% more likely to have initiated sex before the age of 15. Additionally, rural females had more lifetime partners and were more likely to report that they had not used a condom during their last sexual intercourse. Rural African American males showed higher rates of risky sexual behavior than urban males (e.g., a larger percentage had had intercourse and a larger percentage had not used condom during most recent sexual intercourse). However, differences among males in rural and urban communities were not as great as for females in rural and urban communities.

Milhausen and colleagues offer suggestions for why rural youth have higher rates of sexual activity. Rural youth compared to urban youth may see HIV as less of a risk because they encounter fewer HIV-infected individuals. The perception of lower risk is likely to result in fewer protective behaviors. Milhausen and colleagues also cite a study that linked fewer recreational outlets in rural communities to boredom and, subsequently, more problem behaviors (Adimora et al., 2001).

The School as Community

Schools exist within neighborhoods, and social, academic, and psychological well-being of girls is affected by the school environment and their perception of the environment. School environments include teachers and other educators, and these individuals influence girls' academic expectations and achievement as well. School environments in which girls learn separately from boys may also contribute to achievement and expectations.

Teacher's Expectations for African American Girls

A school environment that promotes feelings of discrimination and low expectations from African American girls is not conducive to academic competence. Not only does low teacher expectations and discrimination lower academic performance, they also contribute to other problem behaviors. This is partly because during the period of adolescence, students are especially vulnerable to confirming negative stereotypes. Wong, Eccles, and Sameroff (2003) found that schools in which African Americans feel discrimination from teachers resulted in students engaging in more problem behaviors. Wong and colleagues found that experiences of racial discrimination by teachers were linked to more academic and socioemotional problems. When youth become alienated from school because of perceived discrimination, they are less likely to maintain interest and motivation to do well academically. Perception of discrimination can be reduced by high ethnic identity which may serve as a buffer against discrimination stress. High ethnic identity may alter the trajectory of self-confirming stereotypes as students high in ethnic pride will likely discount stereotypically negative information about African Americans.

In an interesting article titled, "Ladies or Loudies?" Morris (2007) explores how African American girls face unique obstacles related to stereotyping during their educational process. Morris notes that African American girls are not typically seen as problematic as African American boys and are not disciplined as much. However, the author believes that it is possible that African American boys and girls receive differential disciplinary actions in school. He explored this assumption in a 2-year ethnographic study of a public middle school of 1,000 seventh and eighth graders (mostly African American and White with a few Latino students) with approximately 60 educators. Educators were mostly women, African American, and White. The school was located in a poor area of town. For 2 years, Morris was a participant observer; he also interviewed teachers and administered a survey to students. Some of the more interesting findings were: (1) He observed that the African American girls dominated the classroom discussions. Girls tended to be more engaged in answering questions and talked more in science and math classes as well as in English and history classes. Girls were serious about their education and valued academic success. (2) Another observation was that the African American girls stood up to the boys physically. When boys would playfully hit girls, they struck back and did not look to adults for protection. He wrote, "I observed this outspokenness's. Black girls there appeared less restrained by the dominant, White middle-class view of femininity as docile and compliant, and less expectant of male protection than White girls in other educational research." (p. 499). However, he observed that girls' attempts to stand up for themselves with regard to boys did not always meet teacher's approval. (3) He observed that teachers seemed to focus less attention on the academic progress of Black girls. While African American and Latino boys received the most and harshest discipline, African American girls experienced discipline mostly related to the way they acted with teachers believing that they were challenging authority, loud, and not ladylike. Hence the title "Ladies or Loudies?" He observed several examples of Black girls being reprimanded for calling out answers or questioning teachers and saw this less frequently for boys and girls of other ethnic groups. Girls were perceived as too assertive and adult like. Several of the teachers spoke of the girls as being loud and confrontational. Many of the teachers especially the African American female teachers felt that they should help children learn social skills they may not get at home. These included shaping Black girls so that they would display traditionally feminine behavior.

Morris concluded that teachers may have expectations about appropriate feminine behavior based on the norms for White girls. These norms dictate that girls be passive, unassertive, and not talkative. When African American girls do not conform to these expectations, they are disciplined accordingly. This type of interaction and negative reinforcement from teachers can erode self-confidence, limit the girl's voice, and ultimately lower her academic expectations and performance.

Single-Sex Education Classes and Single-Sex Education Schools

Another school context question is whether coeducational or single-sex educational schools and classrooms results in better achievement outcomes for girls. There have been some attempts to evaluate whether single-sex classes are superior to coed classes and schools in academic achievement. However, most of this research has been conducted on White and not African American students. Advocates of single-sex classrooms argue that coeducational environments have unnecessary distractions that get in the way of youth learning. Some have argued that single-sex environments might be especially useful for urban African Americans students as a means in which to increase academic motivation and effort. Findings are mixed, and several studies show no advantages of single-sex schools and classrooms for academic achievement (Singh, Vaught & Mitchell, 1999). Others report that there may be more benefit for girls in single-sex education classrooms than for boys given that research has suggested that girls are given fewer opportunities for classroom participation, are called upon less, and experience more bias from teachers (as the previous study suggested).

Singh & Vaught were interested in whether there were achievement differences in single-sex and coeducational classroom of African American fifth-grade boys and girls in two inner-city schools. Participants were 90 students who attended 4 fifth-grade classes: two were coeducational and two were single-sex classes (both male and female). They found that girls in the single-sex classrooms scored higher than girls in the coeducational classrooms on six out of eight achievement outcomes (e.g., math standardized test scores, science grades, attendance, etc.). The study also found that, overall, girls in the single-sex classrooms seemed to benefit more so than boys in single-sex classrooms. The findings from this study are preliminary due to the small number of classes in the sample, and more research is indicated given the policy implications of single-sex classrooms.

Summary

Communities and neighborhoods have a great impact on the beliefs, values, and actions of girls. Neighborhoods and communities are defined both geographically and socially. In general, research suggests a negative impact of living in disadvantaged, low-resource, and poor neighborhoods. The adverse impact of living in these types of neighborhoods is seen in lower academic expectations and performance, and other problem behaviors such as violence, drug use, and early and risky sexual activity. However, academic achievement among African American girls does not seem to be as affected by living in a poor community as for African American boys.

African American girls who live in poor communities engage in more risky sexual activity than those from more affluent communities. Poor community conditions are also linked to less physical activity, and health problems such as asthma, and drug use. Communities can offer assets and resources. One protective community resource is organizing after-school activities to include recreational activities, clubs, and sports. Girls who are involved in these types of activities are somewhat protected from living in poor communities. Prevention and intervention programs developed and implemented in collaboration with members of the community are likely to be effective and can attenuate the deleterious impact of a disadvantaged community.

Urban communities are often stressful, and stress creates multiple psychological and physical symptoms. Witnessing violence is a stressful event for girls who live in distressed communities, and African American girls tend to experience the harmful effects of this stress more so than boys. Rural communities have their challenges, also, including the lack of recreational activities. Girls from rural communities engage in earlier sexual activity and more risky sexual activity than girls from urban communities.

Schools exist in communities. African American students who perceive discrimination from teachers fare worse academically and also develop other problem behaviors. Teacher expectations about how girls should behave also can result in bias toward African American girls who do not conform to their expectations. Finally, preliminary findings on single-sex classrooms for African American girls show positive academic benefits. However, much more research is needed before we can be conclusive on this subject.

In conclusion, communities and neighborhoods can provide a positive context in which African American girls can thrive socially, academically, and interpersonally. This is true for girls living in both affluent and low-resource communities. To overcome some of the challenges and stressors from living in disadvantaged communities require coordinated efforts among people and the institutions within these communities to provide structure, monitoring, after-school programs, and other prosocial activities.

Recommendations and Resources

Provide Organized After-School Activities in Neighborhoods

Neighborhoods that offer structured and organized after-school activities will promote positive youth development. These activities can range from social clubs to
organized sports to tutoring support. Although girls tend to move away from sports
during adolescence, making sports available to them is still desirable. Organized
and structured activities such as stepping, dancing, and positive hip-hop will likely
appeal to African American adolescent girls.

Provide Mechanisms Wherein Girls Can Contribute to the Beauty of Their Community

After-school programs can provide safe and learning environments for girls while
having them contribute to the community at the same time. Some suggested activities include painting a mural on the wall of a local community-based agency,
planting a garden, and clearing space for a walking trail. This permanent prod-
uct will be a symbol to girls and others in the community of their work and
dedication.

Involve Girls in Volunteer Work and Civic Engagement

The Girl Scouts is a good example of an organization that engages girls in volunteer work and civic engagement. Churches and other religious institutions can also
engage girls in meaningful volunteer work such as cleaning up parks and common
area spaces, visiting nursing homes, and preparing meals in a homeless shelter. Girls
can also be involved in an educational project such as making a documentary on a
topic that is of interest to the community. In our City, teens were involved in making a sex education documentary that was distributed via internet and on compact
discs.

Train a Cadre of Girls Within a Neighborhood to Be Peer Ambassadors for Their Neighborhood

Develop leadership and social skills among girls within a neighborhood on how
to influence other girls and how to model prosocial and positive behaviors. The
training might involve having each girl target her social network of friends within

her community or housing development. Girls could be trained as peer leaders to implement sex and drug prevention programs, and to provide tutoring for younger children.

Use Social Marketing Techniques to Inform the Community

Many communities are now using social marketing techniques to inform residents about the norms for certain problem behaviors such as smoking and drinking. Also social marketing can be used to inform the community about resources and assets in the community. In our local community, prevention messages were displayed on City buses. One of these messages included pictures of girls and their fathers showing the importance of father involvement in their daughter's life. Other messages provided information on resources for addressing problems of community violence, pregnancy, and drug prevention.

Train Teachers in How to Promote Positive Development with Girls

Teachers play an important role in supporting the development of youth. Provide training to school administrators, teachers, and other educators as to how bias against African American girls may be insidious and harmful. Conversely, train teachers in how to promote high expectations, academic achievement, and well-being among girls.

For example, teachers can make sure that boys and girls are called upon with equal frequency and girls should be provided leadership opportunities. Teachers can reinforce that the evaluation of students' work will be based on merit and not gender (Rubenstein & Zager, 2002).

Recommendations from the Institute of Medicine, National Research Council

This report provides recommendations for several ways in which community programs can promote youth development (see Resource section). This report identifies features of community programs that facilitate positive youth development. While these recommendations do not necessarily focus on African American girls, they are beneficial to all youth. Some of these recommendations include:

(a) The environment should be physically and psychologically safe.
(b) The environment should be structured and monitored.
(c) There should be adults with whom youth can develop supportive relationships.

(d) Girls should have opportunities to belong and to feel part of the group.
(e) There should be positive social norms.
(f) Support for developing efficacy and skills should be provided.
(g) The community environment should consider what is happening in the family, and school and lessons learned in these different environments should be integrated and consistent.

Resources

Eccles, J., & Gootman, J. A. (2005). Community Programs to Promote Youth Development. This report is a project of the Board on Children, Youth, and Families within the Division of Behavioral and Social Sciences and Education of the National Research Council, and the Institute of Medicine. The report is available from the National Academies Press at (800) 624–6242 or via the National Academics Press web-site at www.nap.edu

Community Programs to Promote Youth Development: Report Brief: November 2004. Available from: www.iom.edu/Object.File/Master/24/200/FINAL%20Community%20Programs%208-Pager.pdf

Chapter 6
Expectations and Achievement

> *"After I get out of high school, I'm gonna take one year so I can raise some money for me to go to college. After that year, go to college. Four years then I got to go about 9 more years to get my pediatrician degree. Then after that, well during that time, somewhere in between there, I'll probably meet my husband, we get married, and have kids between them nine years..."*
>
> Comments of a teen girl in a focus group to the question, "what are your plans for the future?"

The above quote illustrates the trajectory this teen would use to reach her personal and professional future goals. Children begin to acquire a sense of their future during the period of early to mid adolescence. During this developmental period, they develop hopes, dreams, and aspirations for their future. Life-course expectations influence the goals that girls set for themselves and the actions they choose to reach these goals. If a girl expects to go to college after graduating from high school, her behavior will be directed toward getting good grades and delaying parenthood. If on the other hand, there are no college role models and/or expectations from others for her to attend college, then good grades and academic accomplishment may not be as important.

Life-course expectations are shaped by personal as well as contextual and environmental factors. Parents play an especially significant role in life-course expectations and academic achievement. Parental role modeling (mothers more so than fathers) impact their daughters' life-course expectations with messages that emphasize the importance of finishing school, getting a good job, and delaying parenting. Sometimes parents provide models of what behavior not to emulate in cases where mothers have cut short their education and life goals because of early parenting.

The community and neighborhood in which a girl resides also influences her life-course expectations. Growing up in low-resource and public housing communities tends to be associated with lower life-course expectations for African American girls. In some low-resource communities, there are few role models of success. The typical resident may not have attended college or even graduated from high school and may be unemployed or employed in a low skill jobs. Early parenting may also be normative in low-resource communities. Community influences on behaviors were

F.Z. Belgrave, *African American Girls*, Advancing Responsible Adolescent Development, DOI 10.1007/978-1-4419-0090-6_6, © Springer Science+Business Media, LLC 2009 discussed in the previous chapter but will be explored again in this chapter as it relates to life-course expectations.

This chapter begins with a discussion of academic achievement and provides an overview of differences between African American males and females in academic achievement. Different factors contribute to academic achievement for boys and girls, and these factors are discussed next. This is followed by a discussion of life-course expectations for education, parenting, and marriage. A summary and a "Recommendations and Resources" section complete the chapter.

Academic Achievement

Academic achievement is an important topic because educational attainment has a pervasive influence of all life outcomes, including where we live, what career we choose, and whether we delay parenting and other adult responsibilities. There are differences in the academic achievement of African American males and females, and these differences are discussed next.

The Gender Gap in Academic Achievement

There are racial and gender disparities in academic achievement and these are especially apparent among individuals of low socioeconomic status (Wood, Kaplan, & McLoyd, 2007). For example, the average freshman graduation rate, the percentage of the entering freshmen class graduating in 4 years, is lower for African Americans than any other ethnic group. The average freshman graduation rate for the school year 2004–2005 was the following: African Americans/Black – 60.3; Asian/Pacific Islander – 90.5; White – 80.4; Hispanic – 64.2; and American Indians/Alaskan Natives – 67.2 (National Center for Education Statistics, 2007).

There is a gender difference among African Americans in high school and college graduation rates. High school graduates are those who receive a traditional high school diploma from an accredited high school program. Overall, high school graduation rates are about 77% and about 67% for African Americans (Hechman & LaFontaine, 2007). Graduation rates for African American males are 62% versus 72% for females. Among African American college graduates, females received 66% of bachelor's degrees while males received 34% (Peter & Horn, 2005).

During primary and elementary grades, there are few differences in academic achievement between males and females. However, gender differences in academic achievement began to emerge during early adolescence. Mickelson & Greene (2006) examined academic achievement among second- and eighth-grade African American students. African American male and female second graders did not differ in academic achievement. However, there were differences in test scores among eighth-grade males and females with females scoring higher (Mickelson & Greene, 2006). Academic achievement is influenced by factors such as academic expectations, orientations, and values, and African American girls hold higher academic expectations than boys (Mello & Swanson, 2007). By early adolescence, expectations and perceptions about academic achievement have become internalized as evidenced in test scores, grades, and other performance indicators.

Parents and teachers also contribute to gender differences in academic achievement. Wood, Kaplan, & McLoyd (2007) hypothesized that youth, parents, and teachers would hold lower expectations for male than female students. Their study involved 301 African American caregivers who reported on 466 youth, teachers who reported on 271 youth and 307 youth. Participants in the study completed measures of educational expectations, school environment, and academic achievement. The authors found that teachers and parents held lower expectations with regard to future educational goals for African American boys than girls. Also, boys themselves were less confident about whether they would attend college than girls. These differences remained even when current academic achievement was held constant. That is, expectations were lower among teachers and parents for boys than girls even when boys were doing as well as girls. Teachers had lower expectations for boys than girls at every grade level. The study also found that parents' expectations influenced the relationship between gender and academic expectations. Parents expected about 47% of the males and 61% of females to complete college or beyond. These higher expectations for girls may not exist in other ethnic groups as research suggests in general that boys may have an academic advantage over girls. Also, lower academic expectations for African American males may be due to the fact that historically there have been more noncollege-related careers for males to earn a living in (i.e., military, mechanics, athletics, etc).

Values also account for the difference in achievement outcomes among African American girls and boys as girls may value academic achievement more so than boys. To address this issue, Graham, Taylor, and Hudley, (1998) conducted two studies that examined the achievement values of African American students. In the first study, 304 African American sixth, seventh, and eighth graders were asked to nominate up to three students from their class whom they admired, respected, and wanted to be like. Teachers rated the achievement of each student in the class on a scale. Female students were most likely to nominate high-achieving girls, while boys were more likely to nominate low-achieving male students as people they liked, respected, and wanted to be like.

In a second study, Graham et al. (1998) addressed this same issue, but in this study Latino and White students were included along with African American students. These students were also in grades sixth, seventh, and eighth. Like the first study, these students were asked to provide the names of classmates whom they liked, respected, and wanted to be like. African American girls were more likely to nominate other African American girls, and these girls were more likely to be high achievers. African American girls were least likely to nominate low-achieving classmates as peers they liked, respected, and wanted to be like. Latina and White girls were also similarly more likely to value high-achieving females over average and low-achieving peers. African American males also nominated other African American males over Latino and White male classmates. However, African

American males nominated low-achieving African American boys as the classmates that they liked, respected, and wanted to be like more so than average and high-achieving African American males. Similar findings were found for Latino males whose peer nominations were similar to African American males. However, White males were similar to girls in that they choose high achievers over average and low achievers. The findings from these studies suggest that achievement among African American girls may be similar to that of other ethnic groups; this is not the case with African American boys.

African American males value academic achievement less than females and also view themselves as having lower academic achievement than African American females. Hudley and Graham (2001) presented students of different ethnic groups with hypothetical descriptions of students who displayed high or low levels of achievement and school engagement. The students' task was to select one photograph that they believed matched each hypothetical description from a set of photos of unknown male and female junior high school students from diverse ethnic groups. All the participants most frequently selected photos of ethnic minority males for scenarios of academic disengagement, consistent with cultural stereotypes of these young men. Photos of females across all ethnic groups were selected most frequently for scenarios of achievement strivings.

Educational Expectations

Educational expectations vary for African American girls and boys, and there may be different factors that affect these expectations. In general, African American girls tend to have more optimistic views of their education and careers. They also may possess more career-related skills and competencies (Brown, 1997). One study investigated the long-term educational expectations of African American girls and boys using a national longitudinal sample of 875 young adults who were 2 years beyond high school. Data were also collected when students were in the 8th and 12th grades. Eighth-grade academic performance was the strongest predictor of educational expectation for both African American men and women. Language-related skills were more important in predicting academic expectations for women, and mathematical skills were more important in predicting academic achievement for males. The implication from this study is that early school success is important and that middle school is a critical time for girls to establish the foundation for future educational achievement and performance.

In overview, academic achievement, expectations, and values differ for African American girls and boys with African American girls scoring more favorably on each of these attributes. While there are some racial and ethnic gaps in academic achievement among African American girls and girls from other ethnic group, it appears that African American girls function more similar to girls in other ethnic groups with respect to academic achievement. In contrast, African American males tend to have values, expectations, and academic achievement outcomes that differ from that of males in other ethnic groups (with the possible exception of Latino males). Also, higher expectations and values regarding academic achievement for African American girls are held by teachers and parents. We next turn to some of the factors that may account for these differences.

Factors that Contribute to High Academic Expectations and Achievement

There are several factors that influence academic expectations and achievement. Parents play a significant role in their child's academic expectations and achievement, and children generally follow expectations and achievement of their parents. Community and neighborhoods also contribute to both positive and negative academic outcomes depending upon the type of community. Finally, several personal attributes such as ethnic identity, future orientation, and hope influence expectations and achievement.

How Parents Contribute to Academic Achievement and Expectations

Family and parental attributes such as cohesion, bonding, and monitoring and supervision lead to higher levels of school engagement for girls. Academic achievement is likely to be highest when parents provide both cohesion and monitoring (Annunziata, Hogue, Faw, & Liddle, 2006). The influence of mothers may be especially important to achievement among African American girls. Most African American girls report connections to and feeling close to their family, especially their mothers (see Chapter 3). Perhaps it is this bond that motivates girls to strive for and to be successful in a domain that is valued by mothers.

Mother's level of education may also have an effect on her daughter's achievement. Daughters of more highly educated mothers compared to less educated mothers have higher levels of academic achievement. These mothers are also more likely to help her daughter obtain higher career and educational goals (Kerpelman, Shoffner, & Ross-Griffin, 2002). Parents may influence daughter's academic achievement through shaping her educational orientation and values.

One study investigated how parents impact their children's future educational orientation. Three-hundred-seventy-four African American adolescents in grades 7–12 were included in the study (Kerpelman, Eryigit, and Stephens, 2008). Future education orientation was defined as one's thoughts, dreams, and expectations about what the future holds in terms of educational goals. Kerpelman and colleagues found that perceived maternal support for achievement was related to the student's educational orientation. Parents communicate standards about what their children's educational goals should be, and these in turn influence their educational aspirations. The study by Kerpelman and colleagues also found that mothers had more influence on educational orientation than fathers. Mother support for achievement was a significant factor in educational orientation for both females and males.

A particular style or way of parenting may also facilitate or impede academic achievement among girls. A parenting style that does not provide supervision and warmth may be especially detrimental to academic achievement. Pittman and Chase-Lansdale (2001) conducted a study on parenting style and academic achievement of girls living in poor communities. In this study of 302 African American girls (age: 15–18) and their mother or mother figure, four types of mothers were studied. These included authoritative (mothers who scored high on both warmth and supervision), authoritarian (mothers who scored low on warmth and high on supervision), permissive (mothers who scored high on warmth and low on supervision), and disengaged (mothers who scored low on warmth and low on supervision). Girls whose mothers were disengaged were found to do worse academically than girls whose mothers had one of the three other parenting styles.

How parents racially socialize their children also affects their academic achievement. As discussed previously, racial socialization has to do with how parents socialize or prepare their children to function as an African American in this society. It involves the transmission of values and views about their race and ethnicity (Hughes, 2003). Racial socialization prepares and protects children, and is generally a positive factor in their academic achievement (Neblett, Philip, Cogburn, & Sellers, 2006). Neblett and colleagues were specifically interested in whether racial socialization messages were helpful to academic achievement, especially for those students who perceived that racial discrimination existed. Participants were 548 African American students in grades seven through ten who were recruited from middle and high school. There were 225 males and 323 females in the study. A socialization scale that included several subscales (racial pride, self-development, etc.) was administered along with measures of perceived racial discrimination, academic curiosity, academic persistence, and grades. The authors found that the perception of discrimination was associated with lower levels of academic curiosity, persistence, and grades. Also, measures of self-worth (i.e., positive messages about the self) were related to higher levels of academic curiosity and persistence. In addition, racial socialization messages were correlated with all academic measures. Racial socialization is discussed in more detail in the Chapter 3.

Most of the studies on parental influence on African American children's academic expectations and achievement have been conducted on low-income children and parents who may reside in low-resource communities. However, middle-class parents are also influential to children's academic achievement and expectations. Sirin and Rogers-Sirin (2004) explored this topic with a sample of 336 middle-class African American students and their mothers. Parental influence on academic achievement and other psychological variables was investigated. They found that for this group of African American middle-class students, educational expectations and school engagement had the strongest relationships with academic performance. Their results also indicated that positive parent–child relationships, not parents' educational values, were related to better academic performance. The lack of a positive relationship between students' academic achievement and parental educational values was not consistent with that found in other studies. Other studies have found that parent's educational values along with educational level are important predictors of the academic success of their children. The findings suggest that parental factors are important for middle-class children, but the nature and type of parental influence may differ than for children from lower-status backgrounds. Perhaps factors such as parental values are important as they compensate for other parental resources among students who live and attend school in lower-income communities.

In overview, parental factors affect educational goals, expectations, and achievement. It appears that maternal support is more important and African American mothers have a bigger influence on educational outcomes than fathers (Kerpelman, Eryigit, and Stephens, 2008). Parental expectations and values that promote achievement are important and may be especially beneficial to achievement for girls from lower-income backgrounds.

Ethnic Identity

Ethnic identity is defined and discussed in Chapter 2. Some of the earlier research on this topic suggested that high ethnic and racial pride was correlated with lower academic achievement (Fordham & Ogbu, 1986) among African American youth. The negative relationship between ethnic identity and academic achievement was based on the assumption that academic success is not always rewarded in the African American community; therefore, racial pride may not be affiliated with academic success. Consistent with this is a finding from a more recent study by Neblett and colleagues (2006). These authors found that racial pride messages were associated with lower academic curiosity and grades. The authors speculated that perhaps racial pride messages promote greater anxiety in the classroom which subsequently led to lower engagement and performance.

However, findings from several other studies suggest that ethnic identity promotes academic achievement among African American youth including African American girls (Adelabu 2008; Oyserman, Bybee, & Terry, 2003). Adelabu (2008) investigated the role of ethnic identity (along with hope and future time orientation to be discussed later) on academic achievement in a sample of 661 African American adolescents in grades 7–12. Academic achievement was measured by grade point average. Adelabu found that ethnic identity was correlated with grade point average in the total sample, and the effect was more pronounced for females.

In another study, Kerpelman, Eryigit, and Stephens (2008) examined ethnic identity (along with self-efficacy and perceived family support) and their relation to future education orientation. Their study included 374 African American adolescents who were in grades 7–12. The authors found that females had higher future education orientation scores than males. Ethnic identity was a significant factor in future education orientation for both males and females.

Three components of racial identity might be especially beneficial for African American girls in promoting academic achievement, including: (1) feeling connected to the African American community; (2) being aware of racism; and (3) feeling that achievement is part of being Black (Oyserman, Harrison, & Bybee, 2001). The development of racial identity content transitions from physical attributes (e.g., looking African American) to focusing on skills and competencies of one's racial group. Given this reasoning, Oyserman and colleagues predicted that the relational component of ethnic identity might be more important to boys' academic achievement than the relational component of girls' identity since girls are already relational. They predicted that the belief that achievement is a component of being Black might be especially important for African American girls' academic achievement. Ninety-one-eighth-grade African American students completed a survey with measures of academic efficacy and the three components of racial identity. The authors indeed found a positive relationship between the achievement component of racial identity and academic efficacy among girls in both cross-sectional and longitudinal analyses.

Racial ideological beliefs are related to ethnic identity insofar as they are beliefs about how African Americans should act, think, and behave (Smalls, White, Chavous, & Sellers, 2007). Research supports the positive relationship between racial ideological beliefs and academic achievement among African American girls. In a study of racial ideological beliefs among African American girls, Smalls and colleagues found that beliefs that emphasized being more like Whites, which is an assimilation belief, were related to less academic persistence and more school behavioral problems. Beliefs that emphasized commonalties among African Americans and other oppressed groups (minority ideology) were associated with more positive school engagement. Girls who reported more racial discrimination showed lower school engagement. Girls with strong assimilation beliefs and who reported racial discrimination were especially likely to have low academic identification.

In overview, findings show that strong ethnic identity is a positive factor for academic achievement. This relationship seems to exist more strongly for African American girls than boys. Also, having racial ideological beliefs that encompasses a minority ideology is linked to higher school engagement. Racial discrimination is a risk factor for academic engagement. One's orientation regarding the future is also a factor in academic success and is discussed next.

Future Outlook

Academic achievement is affected by hope and expectations for the future. Future outlook is defined as an individual's thoughts and attitudes about the future (Nurmi, 2004). Detris Honora (aka Adelabu) has conducted quite a bit of research on the topic of future orientation and educational aspirations among African American youth. Educational aspirations are shaped by future outlook as one's future outlook guides academic achievement through long-term goal setting and persistence

(Honora, 2002). Females, in general, tend to set fewer goals and are not as optimistic about their future lives as males, but as with other types of academic outcomes, this is not the case with African American females.

African American teen females are more likely than African American males to have long-term goals and to know how to go about achieving them. Honora (2002) interviewed 16 low-income African American adolescent males and females whose age ranged from 14 to 16. Half were high achievers academically and half were low achievers academically. Participants were asked about their goals and aspirations, their future plans, and what goals and aspirations parents and teachers had for them. Participants reported goals in four categories, including academics, employment, sports, and marriage and family. Girls tended to report more goals than boys in the areas of education, employment, and marriage and family, respectively. Boys reported more goals than girls in the area of sports and leisure.

Honora found that higher-achieving girls provided more goals and expectations than lower-achieving girls and boys. High-achieving girls were also more likely to recognize that major life events should occur in a sequence such as first getting an education, then becoming employed, and then having a family. Lower-achieving girls and boys were more likely to report on goals within a single domain such as employment or academics. For example, these girls reported that they wanted to get a job or complete high school, not both. Lower-achieving girls (and boys) were also less likely to report on future planning and also had more uncertainty about future outcomes. Lower-achieving girls also did not discuss planning a lot and did not feel in control of future outcomes. Finally, higher-achieving students had families who encouraged them and served as models of what to expect in the future. Lower-achieving students tended to not discuss their future goals with their parents or other family members. The findings from this study by Honora suggest that high-achieving girls are likely to set more goals and recognize the temporal spacing of these goals. African American girls are also more likely than African American males to have goals and to understand the relation between present performance and future goals.

One factor that has been investigated in relation to academic achievement is future time orientation. This line of research also suggests that there may be differences in how future time orientation relates to academic achievement for boys and girls. In a study of 616 African American adolescents, Adelabu (2008) found that a future time perspective was predictive of academic achievement for African American girls but not boys. The author reported that African American adolescent males relative to females tended to have more negative expectation for the future and to involve themselves in more short-term planning than long-term planning. Findings from the study by Adelabu suggest that a future time orientation compared to a present or past time orientation may be beneficial for academic success. Given that people of African descent have a cultural value that considers the past and present as well as the future in decision making (Jones, 2003) the topic of time orientation and academic achievement is an important one to address in future research. The Adelabu (2008) study only focused on future time orientation.

The influence of a present and future time orientation was addressed by Adelabu (2007) in a study of 232 African American male and female adolescents who ranged in age from 14 to 20 years. The author was specifically interested in how time perspective was related to feelings of school belongingness and academic achievement and whether females and males differed in this relationship. Among girls, Adelabu found that academic achievement was correlated with a future time perspective. Also, among girls, a present time orientation was negatively associated with academic achievement, and students with a present time orientation tended to report lower grades than those who were less present oriented. Among males, there was also a significant negative relationship among present time perspective and academic achievement. However, future time perspective did not relate to academic achievement among males. These findings show gender differences in these relationships and suggest that factors that motivate academic achievement may differ for African American boys and girls. What seems to be true is that an extended future time perspective encourages girls to set goals and plans for how to carry out these goals.

Hope

A few studies have been conducted on how hope (e.g., a wish with expectation for something) affects academic achievement. Fewer studies have been conducted with African American adolescents and even fewer have involved African American female samples. In general one would expect that students who feel hopeful about their future would be more likely to engage in activities to support future goals. In the study discussed previously by Adelabu (2008), hope was found to be related to academic achievement among the 661 African American adolescents. Hope was a significant predictor of academic achievement for both males and females.

Other Life-Course Expectations

In addition to academic expectations there are other life-course expectations held by African American girls. Life-course expectations, outside the academic domain, are affected by some of the same factors that affect academic life-course expectations, including parents and the community. These include expectations about when to began sexual activity, when to have a baby, when to get married, when to get a job, when to have a career, etc.

What are African American Adolescent Girls' General Life-Course Expectations?

There have been a few studies of life-course expectations among African American girls. In a study of life-course expectations among urban African American teens,

Perez-Febles (1999) involved 166 pregnant and nonpregnant African American adolescent girls and questioned them about their life experiences. She identified two trajectories girls had for family life course. These were "paced" and "accelerated" trajectories. Girls with a paced trajectory, reported an older age at first childbearing, a younger average age at marriage along with an older average age for becoming a grandmother than girls who were in the accelerated trajectory.

Perez-Febles suggests that one must consider the context in which girls live when considering what is normal and what is not normal for African American girls. While adolescent childbearing may be considered undesirable by some, if the teen lives in a community where siblings, friends, and neighbors become parents at a young age, then it is normative and early parenting may be desired.

Linda Burton (2001) studied African American families and found that the average age for becoming a mother in low-resource neighborhoods was 15–18 years, followed by marriage at 28–30, and becoming a grandmother at 34–36. Another study found that the average age for African American women becoming grandmothers was 43.43 years in comparison to 50.1 years for European American women (Watson & Koblinsky, 2000).

With regard to marriage, African American women marry at a lower rate and also at a later age in comparison to White women. The Joint Center for Political and Economic Studies reports by the age of 30, the majority of White women (81%), Hispanic women (77%) and Asian women (77%) will have been married; however, only 52% of Black women will have been married. The socioeconomic conditions and the norms in the communities in which African American girls grow up in may contribute to their expectations for when to marry.

The timing of marital and birth expectations may differ for African American girls than girls from other ethnic groups. East (1998) conducted analysis on timing of sexual intercourse, having a child, and getting married using data collected from 574 girls in seventh and eighth grades. Girls from four ethnic groups (i.e., African American, Latina, White, and Southeast Asian) were asked the best age and the desired age for these first time critical life events. There were several ethnic differences in timing responses. For example, Latina girls reported the youngest desired age for marriage (22.4), and the youngest desired age for birth of first child (23.3). African American girls reported the youngest age for what they believed would be the ideal age of first intercourse (age 19), and they reported the oldest desired age for marriage (24.4). Southeast Asian girls reported the oldest ideal age for first intercourse (21.7) and for first birth (24.3). White girls fell in the middle of the other ethnic groups. The author noted that African American girls compared to girls in the other ethnic groups were least likely to report marriage as important and more likely to perceive that they would have a nonmarital birth. These findings suggest that the expected timing of critical life events differs for African American girls than girls from other ethnic groups. The study by East is over 10 years old, and more recent research on this topic is indicated. However, this finding is consistent with recent data on single female-headed households among African Americans.

Many of the girls who have participated in our programs and research live in communities in which adolescent childbearing is normative and life-course expectations are impacted. In our interviews with African American teen girls, almost all had a friend who was a teen parent if they were not a parent themselves. In these communities, reality shapes expectations and may influence the teen's decisions about when to become sexually active and when to have a baby. Although most of the young girls in our studies report that they will not become sexually active until they are older than 20 years, the average age of actual sexual intercourse is much lower (see Chapter 8).

Girls who have been in our interventions and research have reported high expectations regarding education and careers. When asked what they want to be when they grow up, they report that they want to be cosmetologists, teachers, physicians, and lawyers. Some want to be ministers. While they report fairly high career goals, many do not understand the path that is necessary to reach these goals. For example, several say they want to become a doctor (especially pediatrician), but this takes over 10 years of schooling beyond high school which many girls seem completely unaware of. Clarification of expectations; goal setting; and discussions of education, career, parenting, and marriage options would benefit these girls. These discussions should be throughout childhood and adolescence, but certainly during early adolescence as this is the developmental period in which expectations, goals, and behaviors begin to have a long-term impact on education and career success. These discussions can take place within the home, church, school, and other settings.

The Impact of Poverty on Expectations

Poverty and other economic factors affect girl's life-course expectations and may account for lower life-course expectations among African American girls who grow up in low-resource communities. In an earlier paper, McLoyd & Hernandez-Jozefowicz (1996) discuss how economic hardship factors, socialization factors, and other factors influenced life-course expectancies among 115 seventh- and eighth-grade African American adolescent female students and their single mothers. The sample was considered economically distressed as the majority of the families received aid for dependent children. Daughters were asked how likely it would be that during her adult life she would experience difficulty in finding a good job and supporting herself. Daughters were also asked about the likelihood of having a child without being married, getting married after high school, and getting divorced. Mothers were asked how much concern she held that her daughter would be able to get a good job or would have to depend on welfare. Measures of economic hardship, perception of daughter's academic ability, and educational values were also obtained. The study found that daughters who perceived their families as having economic hardship (i.e., inability to pay for basic necessities) had fewer optimal life-course expectancies. That is, these girls were more likely to believe that their family life course would be characterized by bearing children prior to getting married, by marrying immediately after high school, and by divorce. Mother's level of education also was predictive of daughter's life-course expectations in this study.

Mothers with higher levels of education expected fewer family transitions associated with financial hardship. This is an important study as its findings suggest
that girls' expectations about their future are linked to how they assess the current
economic condition of their family. The authors noted that these girls could be considered more realistic than idealistic. The truth is economic hardship does affect
one's current status and future life expectations.

Career Expectations

Early and middle adolescence is when career interests begin to develop along with
life-course expectations regarding careers. Vocational aspirations and expectations
influence career and vocational choices. Vocational aspirations can be defined as the
desired career goal one has set for herself under ideal conditions (Baly, 1989). Vocational expectations, on the other hand, consider realistic factors that might affect
the attainment of these aspirations (Baly, 1989). Vocational aspirations begin to
develop in early adolescence and become internalized during late adolescence. During this developmental period, adolescents combine information about themselves
with information about available opportunities (Hellenga, Aber, & Rhodes, 2002).
Historical and current contextual factors may affect the vocational and career
expectations of African American girls.

Occupational aspirations provide a sense of what an individual hopes to do,
while expectations provide a sense of what an individual sees herself doing given
her current context. This gap is expected to affect career goals. Hellenga and colleagues studied the career aspiration and expectation gap in a sample of 160 African
American pregnant or parenting adolescent girls (age: 13–19). This group was cho-
sen because they were considered at risk due to financial limitations, and because
they had a baby on the way or a baby that was recently born. Teens were asked
the question, "If you were completely free to choose any job, what job would you
like most as a lifetime job?" to assess their aspirations. To assess expectations, they
were asked, "When you think of your life, what job do you think you will be doing
when you are 30 years old?" Other measures such as economic status, mother's
educational aspirations, perceived support, obstacles to education, and depressive
symptom were also obtained. The study found that the average aspiration level
was significantly higher than the average expectation. However, the majority of the
respondents showed no discrepancy between their aspirations and expectations. The
authors noted also that their beliefs about their vocational futures were more optimistic than might be expected given the disadvantage the girls faced and given her
generally low GPA. The majority of girls expected to graduate from a 4-year college
or from graduate school, and believed they would reach their vocational goals at all
levels of socioeconomic status. Teens with an aspiration-expectation gap had both
higher aspirations and lower expectations than those without a gap at all. We have
seen similar high aspirations and expectations in our work with African American
girls.

In summary, educational aspirations and expectations may be higher for African American girls than their living conditions would suggest. When expectations are high, it is important to have supports and resources in the home and community to support these expectations.

Improving Life-Course Expectations

Since life-course expectations are so important in academic achievement, teen childbearing, careers, and vocations, interventions to improve positive life-course expectations should be beneficial. An example of such an intervention is one on possible selves carried out by Oyserman, Terry, and Bybee (2002). Oyserman and colleagues developed and implemented an intervention that focused on helping youth develop a more detailed view of what their possible or potential self could become. The goal of this intervention was to improve school involvement and academic success by expanding the student's conceptualizations of their possible selves. The sample comprised 208 African American students who were assigned to intervention and comparison groups. Students were in their last year of middle school and resided in an inner city community.

The program used a small group activity format to help participants gain a sense of their vision of their future and to learn how to develop strategies to reach their future goals. The program, called the School to Jobs Program, required students to meet after school for 9 weeks. The study findings showed a positive effect of this intervention on school engagement, school behaviors, and more optimistic possible selves. A more detailed description of this program is in the "Recommendation and Resources" section.

Summary

Life-course expectations are important insofar as they shape goals and behaviors directed at reaching these goals. Life-course expectations regarding education, careers, becoming a parent, and getting married begin to surface during early adolescence and continue in adulthood. Several factors, including both personal and contextual factors, influence these expectations.

African American girls have higher academic performance, aspirations, expectations, and seem to value education more so than boys. Yet, they still lag behind girls from other ethnic groups in terms of academic performance. Ethnic identity, parental support and monitoring, and a future orientation facilitate high academic expectations and achievement among African American girls. Compared to girls from other ethnic groups, African American girls may have lower age expectations for becoming a parent and higher age expectations for getting married. Poverty is a factor in expectations and girls who live in poverty tend to have lower expectations than those who do not.

In conclusion, expectations drive subsequent achievement across all life domains for African American girls. Much can be done to promote high expectations and some suggestions are provided in the next section.

Recommendations and Resources

Increase Expectations and Direct Her Path to Good Career Choices

Provide girls with opportunities to meet people who have different jobs and careers. Host career days in schools, at community forums, and churches. Have girls shadow an employee for a day in a job that she is interested in. Parents can solicit the help of friends, coworkers, supervisors, and others and arrange for their daughter to interview (or shadow) someone in a field that the girl may have voiced an interest in. I have a friend who is an elementary school teacher, and my daughter spent a lot of time when she was in middle and high school hanging out with her and helping her out after school. Prior to her even knowing she wanted to become a teacher, she showed interest in working with younger children (at about the age of 10–11). She also was fortunate enough that her school arranged an internship in this teacher's classroom, and she was able to get some academic credit for it. Thank you Patricia Smith (from Ft. Washington, Maryland). Use supports and other natural resources in the community to encourage her to explore career choices.

Engage in Goal Setting Activities for Short- and Long-Term Plans

Goal setting is an important component of being successful in whatever is achieved in life – education, career, marriage, and parenting. Have girls construct a time line (see later discussion) of what they want to achieve personally and professionally. Discuss both short- and long-term activities to support these goals.

Reinforce the obtainment of short-term goals (doing well on a test, attending a health job fair, etc.). Accomplishing small goals will help her gain confidence in reaching for larger goals and in her overall ability to make good decisions. A good strategy for parents and teachers to use is to ask daughters to set one small weekly goal for herself. Review with her this goal and why it was or was not obtained. Also discuss with her how she felt when she completed or did not complete this goal.

Explore Parental Expectations and Choices for Daughters

This activity should optimally take place in a small group of 5–6 girls and mothers/fathers. Parents are asked to write down what their expectations are for their daughter in terms of her education, career, parenting, marriage, etc. on index cards of one color. Daughters also write down their self expectations for career, education, parenting, on cards of another color. Have parents' cards on one table and daughter's cards on another. See if parents and daughters can find each other's card. This activity provides a good opening discussion of the relationship between parents (especially mother's) expectations and the daughter's life-course expectation. Did parents hold higher or lower expectations than daughters? Were parents' career choices for her daughter more realistic given their circumstance? What were their expectations about childbearing?

Increase Academic Achievement

In the book, *Overcoming the Odds: Raising Academically Successful African American Young Women*, Hrabowski and colleagues (2002) sought to find out the factors that contributed to academic success among African American young adult females. They interviewed college students (and parents) who were enrolled in the Meyerhoff Scholars Program at the University of Maryland, Baltimore County. Women in this program are top students as this competitive program only admits students with very good grades, SAT scores, and with strong science and math backgrounds. The authors conducted interviews with parents and the female students themselves to gain insight into what shaped their high academic performance.

Parental support was a major factor in girls' academic success. Mothers reported that they worked to keep the lines of communication open; used personal experiences to teach lessons with an emphasis on avoiding the wrong crowds; socialized girls to appreciate being Black and female in this country; made their daughters aware of racism and sexism; conveyed the importance of support from family, church, and community; taught them to believe in themselves; and set high expectations for their performance. Fathers of these successful young women wanted to prepare them for life in the real world as well as for academic success. Fathers taught their daughters about men, including the choices and consequences of dating. The female students provided several perspectives on what contributed to her academic success. Some of these included (1) reading at an early age and preference for reading over television; (2) high expectations and encouragement from parents; (3) parental interests in daughter's academic activities such as homework and monitoring of such activities; (4) and involvement in extracurricular activities.

Increase Possible and Positive Self-Expectations

Self-expectations can also be a way to improve academic achievement and other life-course outcomes. An intervention described earlier by Oyserman, Terry, and Bybee, (2002) demonstrated effectiveness for increasing not only school outcomes but also expectations for what is possible. The intervention was implemented during the student's last year of middle school. The intervention used small group activities carried out over nine sessions as follows. (1) The goal of session one was to create a group where there was group cohesion and membership. (2) The goal of the adult image session was to create an image of adulthood, whereby students viewed pictures of adults in different roles and described what they would be like as adults. (3) The timeline goal of the third session was for the students to connect the present with the future by drawing a personal timeline. (4) During the possible selves' session, students graphically mapped out the connection between their present behavior, and what would happen next year, and in their adult life. (5) The goal of the solving everyday problem session was to engage students in solving everyday school-related problems as a group. (6) The sixth session was similar to the previous one but focused on helping participants learn to make plans for the future, including educational plans. (7) In the wrapping up and moving forward session, participants reflected on their experiences in the program thus far and talked about bringing their parents to the group. (8) The goal of the session was to develop communication skills between youth and parents and for parents and students to voice any concerns they had for the coming year. (9) The last session was on jobs, careers, and informational interviewing. This intervention is described in more detail in this paper.

Oyserman, D., Terry, K., & Bybee, D., (2002). A possible selves intervention to enhance school involvement. *Journal of Adolescence, 25*, 313–326.

This intervention could be tailored for African American girls by using female facilitators and convening all girls groups. Session 2, for example, could focus on female adults in different roles. The timeline in Session 3 might include a timeline for parenting and also for marriage. Session 5 might focus on some of the special problems African American adolescent girls face.

Resources

Hrabowski, F. Z., Maton, K. I., Greene, M. L., & Greif, G. (2002). Overcoming the Odds: Raising Academically Successful African American Young Women. New York: Oxford University Press.

Part III

Chapter 7
Health and Wellness

> *"I used marijuana... all the time.... I buy it either me and my*
> *cousins, they buy it and we do it together. I prefer blunts... I use*
> *blunts about four days out of the week."*
> *16-year-old teen mother response to questions about drug use*

What is more valuable than good health? Good health is often taken for granted especially by children and adolescents. However, good health practices, including a nutritious diet and physical activity, instituted during childhood carries over into adulthood. In this chapter, health, wellness, chronic illnesses, and related topics among African American girls are discussed. The chapter begins with definitions followed by a discussion of puberty. Areas of health concern for African American girls include obesity and other chronic health problems, such as asthma and diabetes. Drug use is not as much of a problem for African American girls as for other groups. However, the consequences of drug use are much worse among African American youth, so drug use is discussed along with programs for substance abuse prevention. As illustrated in the quote, drugs such as marijuana, are available. Mental health and psychological well-being is a component of overall health and is also discussed in this chapter. Also included is a discussion of cultural perspective on achieving good mental health.

Definitions

The World Health Organization provides definitions of health and related concepts. Health is defined as a state of complete physical, mental, and social well-being and not merely the absence of disease or infirmity. This definition includes mental and social well-being along with physical well-being. Adolescence is generally a period of good health, particularly physical health. Health habits developed in childhood and adolescence have long-lasting consequences.

Illness can be a symptom for disease or it can be a person's perception of having poor health. Disease is a physiological process that can cause an abnormal condition of the body or mind. A chronic condition is long lasting (e.g., more than 4–6 weeks

F.Z. Belgrave, *African American Girls*, Advancing Responsible Adolescent Development,   109
DOI 10.1007/978-1-4419-0090-6_7, © Springer Science+Business Media, LLC 2009

and in many cases lifelong) and needs to be managed on a long-term basis. Two examples of chronic illnesses discussed in this chapter are asthma and high blood pressure.

Mental health is defined in the Surgeon General's Report on Mental Health (1999) as the successful performance of mental function, leading to productive activities, fulfilling relationships with other people, and the ability to adapt to change and to cope with adversity. Mental illnesses are health conditions that are characterized by changes in thinking, mood, or behavior (or some combination thereof) and are associated with distress and/or impaired functioning. Mental health and mental illness are on a continuum with mental health on one end as "successful mental functioning" and mental illness on the other end as "impaired functioning." No age period brings with it more changes in mental, physical, and social health than puberty which is discussed next.

Puberty

Puberty is the period of human development during which physical growth and sexual maturation occurs, indicating the ability to sexually reproduce (Puberty, 2008). During puberty, there is a growth spurt and physiological, hormonal, emotional, and social changes occur. Physical changes include rapid growth, hormonal increases, and biochemical changes in the brain that affect mood. Psychological changes include increased sensitivity to criticism, mood swings, concern about relationships and friendships, and worries about being unsuccessful. Anxiety and stress becomes more prominent during puberty. Puberty is also the time in which girls begin to develop independence from the family and become more oriented toward relationships outside the home (Negriff, Fung, & Trickett, 2008). Romantic interests begin during this period.

Puberty can begin as young as age 8 for girls and age 10 for boys. However, there is great variation in puberty as will be discussed. Generally, signs of puberty in the United States begin at about age 11 with menstruation occurring two or so years later. At this point, the girl is capable of reproduction. The average age of puberty has declined for all girls in the United States.

The typical ages of initiation for puberty occurs between the ages of 10 and 14 for girls and ages 12 and 16 for boys. African American girls experience puberty earlier than white girls, making their age range for the onset puberty between 9 and 14 (National Institute of Child Health and Human Development [NICHD], 2007). In many cultures, menarche and the outward signs of puberty are celebrated and seen as a welcoming sign of transition to adulthood. However, in this country, puberty is appreciated less. At the other end of the spectrum are girls who have late puberty and menarche. Late puberty have both positive and negative benefits. Sometimes girls who have late puberty do better academically because they channel their energy and activities on academics. However, others may not fit in socially with peers in their age group and may consequently suffer some social isolation.

African American girls tend to enter puberty and menarche earlier than girls from other ethnic groups. Across all girls, the average age of menarche is 12.52 years. For African American girls the average age is 12.06 years, or about a half a year earlier than it is for all other adolescent groups (Anderson & Must, 2005). Higher weight is associated with increased likelihood of having reached menarche.

Because of the earlier age of puberty and menarche for African American girls, they may need support in how to deal with this developmental milestone in a positive way. When puberty and menarche is viewed as a positive symbol of their transformation into womanhood, it helps them to understand and appreciate the privilege and the responsibilities it entails. Dialog and education about her body, reproduction, boys, and relationships must certainly occur at this time if it has not occurred previously (see "Recommendation and Resource" section).

Early Puberty

Girls who began puberty at an age younger than their peers may experience psychological problems such as anxiety and depression (Ge et al., 2003). Also, puberty may adversely affect her social and family relationships. Rapid changes in her body may bring on emotional and psychological reactions that she may not be developmentally ready for. Expectations may also differ for girls in early puberty. The social world often sees here as more mature than she really is. Boys, including older boys, may begin to show interest in her. Her hormonal and biological changes also promote more interest from her in boys and romantic partners.

Ge et al. (2003) examined the effects of early physical maturation and accelerated pubertal changes on symptoms of major depression among 639 African American adolescents. The authors found that for girls, early maturation was consistently associated with elevated levels of depressive symptoms. The authors suggest that the family, including the mother's reaction to her daughter's early physical maturation, can shape how girls react to puberty themselves and may buffer any adverse psychological effects. Parents who talk to their daughters about menarche and physical maturation will likely support her in countering potential negative outcomes from early puberty. Higher body weight contributes to early puberty. Diet and physical activity affect body weight and is discussed next.

Diet and Physical Activity

Diet and physical activity play a significant role in obesity, cardiovascular disease, and other chronic health conditions. There is variation among African American girls but generally their diet is not as healthy as the diet of girls from other ethnic groups nor is their level of physical activity as high.

Diet

Eating habits begin in early childhood. While the diet for most Americans is poor, the diet of teens generally and African American teens more specifically tends to be even worse (Eating disorders information fact sheet: African American Girls, 2008). African Americans are more likely than other ethnic groups to eat fried foods, foods high in fat content, and processed foods such as luncheon meat. Moreover, African Americans do not consume enough high-fiber foods, including fruits and vegetables. High-fat, high-caloric foods, and low-fiber foods contribute to weight gain, obesity, and other medical problems. Other factors that contribute to eating choice include family history and food preferences, cost, and availability of food choices and markets in which food is sold.

Girls model the behaviors and practices of mothers and grandmothers in food preparation and eating habits. Mothers are generally responsible for meal preparation and this dictate the types of meals daughters learn to prepare. One study addressed how preparation of meals could be improved by including both mothers and their teen daughters in a nutritious food preparation program (Stolley & Fitzgibbon, 1997). African American girls and their mothers met weekly for 12 weeks and had follow-up meetings every 3 months for 15 months. Mothers and daughters met separately during sessions. The program introduced them to a low-fat diet and increased physical activity.

The program was culturally congruent and attentive to the African American culture. Sessions were held in a community center within walking distance of the participant's home. Participants brought in their favorite recipes and were shown how to modify these recipes so that they were healthier. The program also considered the availability of foods in the community in which participants lived. Program implementers and participants visited local markets to gain an idea of the availability and cost of foods so that they knew what the participants had to work with.

Other culturally relevant methods and activities, such as dance and music, were used. For example, one activity had participants performing rap songs against fat that were put to music. Another strategy was to give participants magazines targeted to African American women to glean tips and advice.

At the end of the program, mothers' eating habits became consistent with recommended guidelines. Mothers reported eating less fat and also less saturated fats. While the daughters did not change their eating habits as much as their mothers, continued modeling from mothers likely helped them to have better food choices in the long term.

The developers of the program recognized that accessible and availability of foods may be problematic in low-income communities. Low-income communities often do not have large chain supermarkets in which to make more economical and nutritious food selections. Small markets in many low-income communities have fewer selections of fresh fruits and vegetables. Farmers' markets and local wholesale food suppliers are almost nonexistent in low-income communities. Yet, better food choices are still possible.

Cost is another factor. Fresh fruits and vegetables and nonprocessed foods are more expensive than processed foods. Four members of Congress took up the pledge to eat for a week on $21. This is the same amount an average food stamp recipient receives. Rep. Jim McGovern (D-Mass.) and Rep. Jo Ann Emerson (R-Mo.), cochairmen of the House Hunger Caucus, encouraged lawmakers to take the "Food Stamp Challenge" to raise awareness of hunger and what they believed to be inadequate benefits for food stamp recipients (Congressional Food Stamp Challenge, 2007).

McGovern and his wife, Lisa, did their food shopping for the week with some tips from a food stamp recipient. In spite of these tips, McGovern reported that it was still a struggle. "No organic foods, no fresh vegetables, we were looking for the cheapest of everything," McGovern said. "We got spaghetti and hamburger meat that was high in fat – the fattiest meat on the shelf. I have high cholesterol and always try to get the leanest, but it's expensive. It's almost impossible to make healthy choices on a food stamp diet."

There is no easy solution for healthy food choices when the budget is inadequate. Yet, creative ways of addressing healthy food choices can be made by families who work together to come up with solutions. Essential vitamins and minerals also contribute to health and these are discussed next.

Vitamins and Minerals

Studies have reported that African Americans are more likely to be deficient in micronutrients. A micronutrient is a vitamin or mineral obtained from outside sources and is not manufactured by the body. Low micronutrient intakes may lead to long-term health risks, especially among African Americans who may be at higher risk than other ethnic groups for developing cardiovascular diseases such as hypertension. The combination of micronutrients such as calcium, magnesium, potassium, as well as folate may be beneficial for blood pressure (Affenito et al., 2007). Antioxidants and vitamin D may modify cardiovascular disease risk as well by maintaining vascular function and health.

Affenito et al. conducted a study to examine whether the presence or absence of benefits from multivitamin/mineral supplements could be used to prevent cardiovascular disease. They examined micronutrient intake in a large sample of African American and White girls from childhood through adolescence (age: 9–18 years). The researchers found that overall White girls tended to consume greater amounts of micronutrients compared to African American girls, with the exception of vitamins E and C, and zinc. For all girls, intake of vitamins A, D, and C; calcium; and magnesium tended to decrease across the years.

The rate of decrease for vitamin D, calcium, and magnesium was greater among African American girls. Moreover, there were ethnic differences in intake trends over time for vitamins E, B-6, B-12, folate, and zinc, which typically increased for White girls but remained stable or decreased among African American girls. The researchers suggest that improving the diet to meet the nutrient reference standards may be an effective approach for reducing cardiovascular disease risk especially among African American girls.

Fitness and Physical Activity

Physical activity declines during adolescence for all girls. This is in part due to increased interests in nonphysical activities, more time spent with peers, after-school employment, and other responsibilities. Gender role beliefs about appropriate physical activity for males and females may also contribute to girls becoming less interested in activities that they may have done previously such as basketball, bicycling, running, etc.

While there is a substantial decline in physical activity among both African American and White girls during adolescence, the greatest decline occurs among African American girls. Kimm and colleagues, (2002) found that by ages 16 or 17, 56% of African American girls and 31% of White girls report that they have no regular physical activity during leisure time.

One of the reasons African American girls report that do not want to participate in physical activities is because they do not want to "sweat." Related to this are concerns about hair. As African American girls reach adolescence, a fair amount of time and effort is spent on making sure their hair looks good. Physical activity, especially activity involving perspiration and water, will undo all the work that has gone into a good hair do. One African American adolescent girl I know preferred to receive a failing grade in a physical education class rather than get her hair "messed up." Fortunately, more versatile hair styles (e.g., braids, natural hair styles, some weaves, etc.) are available so that hair is not as much a barrier to participating in physical activity. Also, physical activities such as dancing and stepping may be more engaging and fun for African American compared to activities such as running and swimming. Poor diet and the lack of physical activity are contributors to some of the chronic health problems discussed next.

Chronic Health Conditions

Chronic health problems that begin in childhood and adolescence are linked to a host of other more serious and sometimes life-threatening medical problems later in life. Prevention is important in keeping these conditions from surfacing in the first place. Obesity is one condition that is of major concern among African American girls.

Obesity

Obesity is defined by body mass index. Obesity is also defined as being 20% above ideal weight as determined by height and/or body mass index. The National Health and Nutrition Examination Survey (Center for Disease Control [NHANES], 2006) indicated that over the past 10 years, adolescents have increasing in being overweight from 11% to 17%. Data have shown that 25% of African American girls, from the ages of 6 to 17, are considered overweight in comparison to 16% of White (non-Hispanic) girls and 17% of Mexican American girls (Federal Interagency Forum on Child and Family Statistics, 2007).

Prior to puberty, African American girls are leaner than White girls, but during adolescence, differences begin to emerge between the two groups (Nainggolan & Murata, 2007; Kim & Glynn, 2004). Puberty brings with it a significant gain in fat tissue for both African American and White teens, but a larger gain for African Americans. At age 9, there are no ethnic group differences in adiposity (also known as fat tissue). However, adiposity for African American girls became significantly greater at age 12. For each chronological age, there is a greater accrual of adiposity in African American girls, because they mature earlier than white girls.

The reasons for obesity are varied and complex. Both life style and genetic factors contribute to obesity. Parents who are obese are more likely to have obese children, due to both genetics and life style factors. Lack of exercise and physical activity, including not being able to go outside because of unsafe conditions in one's neighborhood, are other contributing factors. Diets which include few fruits and vegetables, and whole grains are other factors. Oversized portions, fast foods, and foods high in unhealthy fats are still other contributing factors for obesity.

Gordon-Larsen and colleagues (2004) conducted a qualitative study of 12 African American girls and their maternal caregivers. The purpose of the study was to understand household and physical environmental barriers to physical activity. Gordon-Larsen found that girls preferred sedentary rather than active activities. Also, caregivers were not unaware of the amount of time their daughters spent watching television and believed watching television benefited them by providing supervision. Other barriers to physical activity included lack of affordable and accessible recreation facilities.

Obesity increases the risk of hypertension, other cardiovascular disease, and diabetes. Also, social isolation and stigma may occur with obesity. While African American adolescents are more likely to accept a larger body size than adolescents from other racial and ethnic groups (Kelly, Wall, & Eisenberg, 2005), those who are obese still face stigma. Overweight and obese teens are more likely to be isolated and lonely than those who are not. During early adolescence from about 11 to 13, the stigma and social isolation associated with obesity is greatest.

The Girls Health Enrichment Multisite Studies (GEMS) program, funded by the National Institute of Health, was developed to focus on the prevention of excessive weight gain in African American girls as they enter and proceed through puberty (Rochon et al., 2003). This multisite program field tested several strategies to deal with the problem of obesity among African American girls. Girls 8–10 years of age were eligible to participate as the investigators wanted to intervene with girls prior to puberty. The program tested several interventions. For example, one study targeted African American girls and one of her parents. The intervention promoted healthy eating habits and improved physical activity (Klesges et al., 2004). Another project labeled "fun, food, and fitness," involved girls in a 4-week summer day camp followed by an 8-week home internet program. The findings from the GEM studies have shown overall positive gains in fitness and dietary practices (Baranowski et al., 2003).

Diabetes

Diabetes is a condition in which the level of glucose (sugar) in the blood is too high. The body is unable to convert food into energy resulting in higher-than-normal blood sugar levels. African American children have lower rates of Type 1 diabetes than White children. However, the prevalence of Type II diabetes which develops generally after age 40 is higher among African American children (National Institute of Diabetes and Digestive and Kidney Diseases, 2007). Type II diabetes is linked to obesity and life style factors such as physical activity. One in four black women, 55 years of age or older, has diabetes and diabetes is the third leading cause of death among African American women. Furthermore, it is estimated that close to 15% of all African American over the age of 20 have diagnosed and undiagnosed diabetes. Many African American girls will see their mothers, aunts, grandmothers, friends, and others with diabetes at some point in their lives.

In fact, African American girls may be at risk for diabetes. Young-Hyman and colleagues (2001) investigated hyperinsulinemia or insulin resistance as a risk factor for future type 2 diabetes among 5- to 10-year-old overweight and obese children. The study found that African American girls, in particular, show evidence of insulin resistance in response to a glucose load, suggesting that the early stages of metabolic decomposition that lead to type 2 diabetes may occur at a young age. Young-Hyman recommended that monitoring of insulin resistance should become part of routine medical care for overweight or obese African American children.

Asthma

Asthma is a chronic illness characterized by inflammation of the air passages resulting in the temporary narrowing of the airways that transport air from the nose and mouth to the lungs. Asthma symptoms can be caused by allergens or irritants that are inhaled into the lungs, resulting in inflamed, clogged, and constricted airways. Symptoms include difficulty breathing, wheezing, coughing, and tightness in the chest (Asthma and Allergy Foundation of America, 2008). Asthma attacks can vary from mild to life-threatening. Many factors can trigger an asthma attack, including allergens; infections; exercise; abrupt changes in weather; or exposure to airway irritants, such as tobacco smoke (National Center for Health Statistics [NCHS], 2004). Asthma is the most common chronic condition among children (National Academy on an Aging Society, 1999).

African Americans have the highest asthma prevalence of any racial/ethnic group. The current asthma prevalence rate among African Americans is 36% higher than that for Whites (NCHS, 2004: National Health Interview Survey [NHIS],

2004). African American women have the highest asthma mortality rate of all groups, and mortality is more than 2.5 times higher than for White women (National Institute of Allergies and Infectious Diseases, 2001). Racial disparities also exist in treatment for asthma. African American children are three times more likely to be hospitalized for asthma and more than four times likely to die from asthma (Akinbami & Schoendorf, 2002).

Although asthma prevalence is higher for women than men, boys have a higher asthma prevalence rate than girls. Prevalence for boys is about 68/1,000 compared to 47/1,000 prevalence for girls (Akinbami, 2006). Given these health disparities, it is important that parents of African American children and adolescents learn to manage asthma by seeking treatment and limiting exposure to environmental conditions that contribute to asthma.

There are also ethnic differences in parent perception of asthma (Wu, Smith, Bokhour, Hohman, & Lieu, 2008). Parents of children with persistent asthma enrolled in a Medicaid health plan were interviewed about their children's expectations for functioning with asthma. African American and Latino parents had lower expectations for their children's functioning with asthma, higher levels of concern about their children's asthma, and more competing family priorities compared to White parents (Wu et al., 2008). These parents concerns seem justified given health disparities for African American youth. We turn our attention to mental health issues next.

Mental Health

Mental health is not just the absence of mental illness but the presence of well-being and satisfaction in life. Positive family and peer relationships and purposeful and meaningful activity within the school and community contribute to good mental health.

Certain personality attributes and values also support good mental health. Self-esteem and self-worth are two such factors that are important to mental health as are accomplishments and feeling of control. Some of the more serious mental health disorders include depression, anxiety, and mood disorder.

Mental health problems are likely to surface during adolescence. During adolescence, change is inevitable and with change comes doubt, fears, and sometimes negative appraisal of the self. These fears can lead to depression, anxiety, and self-destructive behaviors such as drug use and risky sexual behavior. Depression is discussed next.

Depression

Depression is one of the most common mental health problems among adolescent girls (Franko et al., 2005). Overall girls have an incidence of depression that is two to three times greater than for boys (Broderick & Korteland, 2002). Girls seem to experience an increase in depression sometime between the ages of 13 and 15.

Franko and colleagues (2005) conducted a longitudinal study of ethnic differences in depression among 1,727 African American and White girls between the ages of 16 and 18. They obtained information from teens 3 years later. The authors found that among White girls depression scores decreased over time, whereas among African American girls depression scores stayed consistent (Franko et al., 2005). The authors speculate that there may be ethnic differences in risk factors for the two groups. For example, the decrease in depression among White girls may be due to the fact that White girls who are depressed may be more likely than African American girls to receive treatment. African American girls who are depressed may not be as likely to receive treatment.

Concerns over body weight have been noted as a contributor to depression among adolescent females. However, body weight as a stressor for depression is not equally distributed across all ethnic and racial groups. African American girls (more so than girls in other ethnic groups) are generally more satisfied with their bodies and thus may be less vulnerable to experiencing depression as a result of weight concerns (Granberg, Simons, & Gibbons, 2008).

Cultural Factors in Mental Health

African American cultural values such as communalism, ethnic identity, and spirituality are linked to positive mental health for African American girls. Studies have shown that high ethnic identity, i.e., feelings of belongingness and connections to one's racial and ethnic group, promotes good mental health (Corneille, Ashcraft, & Belgrave, 2005; Woods & Jagers, 2003). Spirituality and religious involvement are also associated with positive mental health (Goldston, Molock, & Whitbeck, 2008; Le, Tov, & Taylor, 2007). Constantine, Alleyne, Wallace, and Franklin-Jackson (2006) studied the relationship between Africentric cultural values and life satisfaction among a sample of 147 African American girls. The authors found that having more Africentric cultural values were associated with higher levels of self-esteem and social support satisfaction. Higher levels of self-esteem in turn were linked to greater life satisfaction. As discussed in previous chapters, cultural values also provide a buffer against stressors arising from racism, sexism, and discrimination.

Drug Use

Being African American and female reduces the likelihood that a girl will use drugs. African American and Asian girls consume tobacco, alcohol, and other drugs less than girls from other ethnic groups (Wallace et al., 2003). Among 12th graders in 2000, 27% of White girls, 5.1% of African American girls, and 10% of Asian girls reported daily cigarette smoking. This same survey reported heavy alcohol use in the previous 2 weeks as 28.3% for White girls, 8.3% for African American girls, and 11.1% for Asian girls. Marijuana use was 20.8% for White girls, 12.7% for African American girls, and 9.1% for Asian girls.

While drug use is lower among African American girls than girls from other ethnic groups, there are still reasons for caution. African American teens and young adults have far worse consequences from drug use than teens from other ethnic groups. Drug use among African Americans is associated with more severe personal, social, and health consequences (Wallace & Muroff, 2002). Drug use also tends to escalate more rapidly between adolescence and young adulthood for African Americans (SAMHSA, 2002). Girls who use drugs are also more likely to engage in unprotected sex and are subsequently at risk for sexually transmitted diseases and pregnancy. They also are at higher risk for becoming victimized.

For these reasons and others, we want to prevent drug use before it starts. Girls often begin to use drugs because of relationship needs and demands. In Chapter 2, we discussed the importance of relationships to girl's sense of self. Wanting to please others, to not be alone, and to fit in are factors that contribute to drug use among girls more so than boys. Boyfriends, especially older boyfriends, are often the person who introduce girls to drugs. Also, girls are more likely to obtain their drugs in the home from older siblings, relatives, and friends.

Societal factors such as racism also contribute to smoking and drug use among African American girls. Guthrie and colleagues (2002) conducted interviews with African American female adolescents. Participants were asked questions about substance use and their perception of racial discrimination along with other questions. The majority of the girls reported that they had experienced racial discrimination. Their perceptions of everyday racial discrimination were strongly associated with their smoking habits.

Some of the factors that keep girls from not using drugs include positive relationship with family, good academic performance, and feeling good about herself (Clark, Belgrave, & Nasim, 2008). Being connected to a non drug-using peer group, and having positive racial and ethnic identity also protects girls against drug use (Belgrave, Brome, & Hampton, 2000; Townsend & Belgrave, 2000). We have implemented prevention programs that have increased these cultural attributes among African American girls.

Our drug prevention programs have targeted African American girls in early adolescence as this is the age in which tobacco, alcohol, and other drug use is likely to begin (Belgrave, Reed, & Plybon, 2004). Our programs consider both the culture of being a girl and African American and also the skills needed to resist drugs. For example, we discuss the impact of drugs on the African American community, how African Americans are stigmatized in the media with regard to drug use, and how the decision to use drugs is counter to the overall good of her family and other significant others. Activities to strengthen ethnic and racial identity and positive gender roles and relationships are implemented so that positive feelings about self and ethnic and cultural group increase. We used African proverbs to introduce girls to the danger of using drug (e.g., "when the cock is drunk, he forgets about the rooster").

At the same time, girls learn the skills to refuse drugs when drugs are offered. They learn about the effects of drugs on the body, the consequences of using drugs, and how to resist peer pressure to use drugs. In an evaluation of this approach, girls who participated in our culturally adapted drug prevention intervention increased in drug refusal efficacy more so than those who were in a comparison group (Belgrave et al., 2004).

Recognizing the importance of mothers in preventing drug use, Schinke et al. (2006) developed and implemented an intervention for African American mothers and daughters. The intervention focused on interpersonal relationships, positive communication, and respect between girls and their mothers. The intervention consisted of five modules that were delivered via a CD-ROM. The content used animated graphics and voice-over narrative and characters that portrayed an urban Black adolescent girl and her mother. Eighty-six African American and Caribbean American adolescent girls and their mothers participated in the study. Girls' age ranged from 9 to 12. Half of the girls and their mothers were in the intervention group and half were in a comparison group. The findings showed significant gains for girls in the intervention group in terms of improved communication and feelings of closeness with their mothers at posttest. Mothers also reported more positive communication with their daughters and feeling closer at posttest. Poor family communication and conflict is a risk factor for substance use, and this intervention is promising for decreasing risk and increasing protective factors. In overview, drug use has serious and negative consequences for African American girls and programs and activities to deter girls from using drugs are necessary.

Summary

Health is a state of complete physical, mental, and social well-being and is not merely the absence of disease or infirmity. Many changes occur during puberty, including changes in physical, social, and psychological status. African American girls experience puberty earlier than girls from other ethnic groups, and this early puberty may bring about some adverse social and psychological reactions. But good communication and support from her family can buffer African American girls who experience early puberty.

African American girls have less healthy diets and also less physical activity when compared to girls from other ethnic groups. Poor diet and the lack of physical activity contribute to greater prevalence of obesity and diabetes among African American girls. Asthma is another chronic health condition that disproportionately affects African Americans children and adults. Depression affects a fair number of adolescent girls, including African American girls, and is also a health concern. Cultural attributes such as ethnic identity, communalism, and spirituality have been associated with less depression and better mental health. While African American girls use drugs less than girls from other ethnic groups, the consequences are worse. Culturally tailored drug prevention programs for African American girls have been effective in increasing drug refusal efficacy.

Although this chapter has focused on adverse health outcomes among African American girls, most experience good health. The focus therefore should be on establishing good health habits to maintain good health and to prevent disease and disability. Some strategies are reviewed next.

Recommendations and Resources

The activities, exercises, and discussion topics that follow can be used to enhance African American girl's overall health and fitness. Additional activities related to mental health can be found in Chapter 2 on self and identity.

Increasing Good Food Choices and Nutrition

The objective of these exercises and activities is for girls to learn how to make better food choices. There are several good web sites on food, physical activity, and disease prevention. Some are provided in the "Resource" section.

Shopping for Low-Cost Nutritious Food

Have girls make a shopping list based on a fixed budget. The budget of $21.00/per person/week that food stamp recipients get is a good one to start with. Take the group to a local grocery and purchase foods off the list. Convene the group and discuss one or more of the following: (1) how to read the label; (2) what food choices are healthy choices; and (3) what food choices are not healthy. Encourage the girls to share what they learn with their family.

Preparing African American Dishes

Have girls identify dishes prepared by members of their families that they especially like. They should list the ingredients that comprise the dish and get the recipe from a parent or family member. Have the girls prepare the dish at home so that it has less fat and calories and uses more nutritious ingredients. Encourage them to find healthier substitutes for some of the ingredients (e.g., unsweetened apple sauce can be used in place of oil, olive oil can be used to season food rather than animal fat, etc.). If this activity is a group activity, have them bring a dish for all to sample.

Discuss the Significance of Food Within the African American Family and Community

Food is a ritual in most African American homes and food symbolizes both celebratory accomplishments and sad times (witness the extensive food display prior to and after a funeral). Recognizing that preparation and eating of food is a ritual that African Americans have been socialized to from birth allows program implementers to understand the significance of food within African American families and communities. Program implementers can discuss how to honor this ritual in a healthy way.

Involve Mothers and Other Family Members in Nutrition Programs

Nutrition programs that involve mothers and other family members are more likely to be effective than those that just involve youth alone. Mothers are likely to be the person most responsible for purchasing food items and preparing meals. Create opportunities for mothers and daughters to attend cooking demonstrations together. Encourage them to prepare dishes that taste well and are healthy.

Increasing Physical Fitness and Activities

Fitness Activities Should Be Culturally Relevant

Fitness activities should be ones that are culturally engaging. Use of positive hip-hop music and fitness activities such as dancing and stepping may be more engaging than swimming and other types of activities.

Resources

The U.S. Department of Agriculture contains information about steps that can be taken to maintain a healthy weight. The website has links to appropriate food groups, food portions, nutrient-packed foods, and how to use physical activity in achieving a healthy weight. The address is: http://www.mypyramid.gov/steps/stepstoahealthierweight.html

The U.S. Department of Agriculture also has a website for parents and caregivers. The site provides information that helps parents make smart eating choices as well as how to maintain an active lifestyle in order to be good models for children. Resource includes sample menus and how fun and exercise can be incorporated into family play time. The web address is: http://www.fns.usda.gov/eatsmartplayhardhealthylifestyle/Default.htm

The Office of Women's Health has a web site for girls between the ages of 10–16. This site provides information to help girls learn about health and related topics including fitness, nutrition, drug and alcohol, and relationships. http://www.girlshealth.gov/

Chapter 8
Sexual Behavior and Consequences

"I think they don't really know what they are getting themselves into. Because it's more than pleasure, it's a lot of things that go along with that ... I think it's a negative experience for them—it's negative because they don't need to be experiencing that, at that age, and it's negative because if they become pregnant, or if they catch something behind that, it's going to become very negative, and it's not worth that chance."

A teen's response to question "do you know a girl who is having sex and if yes, how do you think she feels about it?"

Teen sexual behavior and related topics have been extensively discussed by the general public and studied by researchers. Topics have ranged from frequency and types of sexual activity, adolescent pregnancy and parenting, to sexually transmitted infections and HIV. African American girls have also been the subject of these discussions and studies. As the quote illustrates, girls themselves are aware of the negative consequences of having sex. In fact, a girl's sexual decisions affect almost every aspect of her life from relationships with her family, to health and well-being, to academic and career success. Early and unprotected sexual activity leads to several adverse outcomes, including pregnancy and parenting, HIV, and other sexually transmitted infections. Sexual activity at a young age also contributes to depression and anxiety and impaired relationships with family and friends. Other consequences include disrupted schooling and limited career options when teens, especially young teens, have unplanned births. In this chapter, sexuality and consequences are discussed. The chapter begins with definitions of sexuality and related concepts. Statistics on sexual activity of African American girls are then presented, followed by a discussion of pregnancy and parenthood. Factors that contribute to early and risky sexual activity are then reviewed.

F.Z. Belgrave, *African American Girls*, Advancing Responsible Adolescent Development,   123
DOI 10.1007/978-1-4419-0090-6_8, © Springer Science+Business Media, LLC 2009

Definitions

Sexuality is the state of being a sexual being. It involves intimacy and a desire to be with a romantic partner. Sexual acts include sexual intercourse, oral and anal sex among, other intimate acts. The Merriam-Webster dictionary defines sexual intercourse as "heterosexual intercourse involving penetration of the vagina by the penis." Sexual behavior is considered risky when it occurs outside of a mutually mono, relationship without condom use, with multiple partners, and/or with partners who are at high risk such as partners who are intravenous drug users and with men who have sex with men.

The adverse effects of teen sexual activity are most pronounced when sex occurs at an early age. Early sexual activity is defined as sex that occurs among teens who are 13 years or younger. Teens at this young age often lack the emotional and cognitive capacity to make good sexual decisions around partner choice, and condom and other contraceptive use. Sexual activity among youth in the United States, including African American teens, is discussed next.

Sexual Activity Among African American Teen Girls

Data collected from the Youth Risk Behavior Surveillance (YRBS) Survey indicate that African American teens, both males and females, have higher levels of sexual activity than teens from other ethnic and racial groups (CDC, YRBS, 2008). The YRBS Survey is a national survey conducted by the Centers for Disease Control that gathers information on sexual activity and related behaviors among youth. Students from public and private schools in grades 9–12 in the 50 states and the District of Columbia respond to questions about sexual activity and other risk behaviors.

The findings from the YRBS survey show that nationwide 47.8% of students have had sexual intercourse at least once during their lifetime. More African American (66.5%) than White (43.7%) and Hispanic (52%) students had engaged in sexual intercourse. The prevalence of sexual intercourse was higher among African American female (60.9%) than White female (43.7%) and Hispanic female (45.8%) students. There was also a higher prevalence among African American male (72.6%) than White male (43.6%) and Hispanic male (58.2%) students.

The YRBS survey also reports on the number of students who have engaged in sexual intercourse with one or more persons during the 3 months preceding the survey. These students are considered currently sexually active. The national prevalence of students who were currently sexually active was 35%. The prevalence of current sexual activity was higher among African American (46%) than White (32.9%) and Hispanic (37.4%) students. The prevalence was higher among African America female (43.5%) than white female (35.1%) and Hispanic female (35.3%) students. And the prevalence was higher among African American male (48.7%) than white male (30.6%) and Hispanic male (39.6%) students.

Despite the higher rates of sexual activity among African American girls, there has been a decline in prevalence of sexual activity. For example, over a 10-year period, the trends in sexual activity among African American girls declined from 65.6% in 1997 to 60.9% in 2007. Not all African American girls are sexually active and some of the reasons why some are abstinent will be discussed along with factors that promote and inhibit early and risky sexual activity. African American teens are also more likely to initiate sex at a younger age and this is discussed next.

Age of Initiation

About 7% of students in the 9th–12th grade report that they had sexual intercourse for the first time before age 13 years (CDC, YRBS, 2008). The rate of early sexual initiation is 6.9% among African American girls, 4.5% among Hispanic girls, and 2.9% among White girls. The rate of early sexual activity is also higher among African American males at 26.2% compared to Hispanic males (11.9%), and White males (5.7%).

Does this mean that African American girls are less responsible and casual about sex than teens from other ethnic groups? This is not necessarily the case as we will see next. For example, sexually active African American teens report more condom use than other ethnic groups.

Contraception and Condom Use

Contraception and consistent use of condoms prevent pregnancy and decrease the risk for sexually transmitted infections. Among currently sexually active students nationwide, 61.5% reported that either they or their partner had used a condom during last sexual intercourse (Centers for Disease Control, 2008). More sexually active African American teens reported using a condom than teens from other racial and ethnic groups. Condom use during last sexual intercourse was higher among African American females (60.1%) than White (53.9%) or Hispanic females (52.1%). Condom use was also higher among African American male (74%) than White (66.4%), or Hispanic (69.9%) male students.

In fact, condom use has increased among African American high school students over the past 15 years. Only about 48% reported using condoms in 1991 in contrast to 67.3% who reported using condoms in 2007. Today condoms are more accessible, there is less stigma and embarrassment associated with condom purchase, and HIV prevention messages encourage condom use.

However, many teens still perceive male condom use as an act that should be initiated by males in sexual encounters. This is true even among older African American teens and adults. We implemented an HIV prevention program for young African American adult females (age: 18–31), many of whom were in college (Belgrave et al., 2008). Most of these women reported that they had purchased condoms and carried condoms on their person. But few had initiated a discussion about condom use and even fewer knew how to put a condom on their partner. Girls in early adolescence have even less experience with discussing condoms and putting condoms on male partners. Similarly, many girls and young adult females have little knowledge of or experience with female condoms.

While African American girls use condoms with higher frequency than girls from other racial and ethnic groups, they do not use birth control pills as frequently. The prevalence of having used birth control pills before last sexual intercourse was higher for White females (24%) than African American females (12.1%) and Hispanic females (9.1%) students. It was also higher among the female partners of White male (17%) than African American male (6.3%) and Hispanic male (9.0%) students (Centers for Disease Control, 2008).

Risk and Protective Factors for Early and Risky Sexual Activity

Teen sexual activity and pregnancy have been topics of discussion and research by the general public and the scientific community for decades. Individual-level factors such as puberty and self-esteem as well as external factors (e.g., peers, school, and community context) play a role in sexual behavior. These factors may contribute to encouraging girls to make responsible sexual choices (i.e., delaying sex, limiting partners, using condoms). Conversely, these factors may contribute to poor sexual choices (early sexual activity, multiple partners, sex with older males, and noncondom use). One biological factor that contributes to sexual initiation is puberty.

Puberty

Puberty was discussed in the previous chapter and is revisited in this chapter with regard to sexual behaviors. Girls typically begin puberty between the age of 9 and 13. During this period, girls experience physical, hormonal, and sexual changes and become capable of reproduction. Puberty also brings rapid growth and the appearance of secondary sexual characteristics such as breasts and pubic hair. The start of puberty brings with it an increased interest in sex. Puberty is also accompanied by changes in social, emotional, and family conditions that sometimes interact with puberty to place girls at risk for poor sexual choices. For example, family conflict (discussed in Chapter 3), a risk factor for early and risky sexual behavior, might increase as girls mature. Family conflict might be brought on by the teen's attempt to gain independence which might be viewed by parents as oppositional.

Although we are not sure of all the reasons, African American girls reach puberty before girls of other ethnic groups. By their ninth birthday, 48% of African American girls and 15% of White girls show clear signs of puberty (e.g., breast development, pubic hair). Menarche occurs during the age of 11 for 28% of African American girls and 13% of White girls. At age 12, 62% of African American girls and 35% of white girls have started menstruating (Herman-Giddens et al., 1997). Because African American girls reach puberty before girls in other racial and ethnic groups, this might partially account for increased sexual activity. Social and psychological factors also affect sexual initiation as discussed next.

Self-Worth and Self-Image

As discussed in Chapter 2, how a girl feels about herself and her image has a profound impact on her functioning in many of life's domains. In no domain is this relationship more clearly seen than in the sexual domain. Numerous studies have shown a link between low self-worth, poor self-image, and early and risky sexual activity (Laflin, Wang, & Barry, 2008; Salazar et al., 2004). Teen girls may enter into sexual relationships because of low self-esteem and self-worth believing that a male partner will provide the love and assurance they need to feel good about themselves. Within this relationship, sex may be perceived as a way to obtain and maintain desired social and emotional connections. These beliefs also contribute to early parenting (to be discussed later).

Sexual Abuse

Girls who have been sexually abused are especially likely to have low self-esteem and are at elevated risk for early and unprotected sexual activity (Goodkind, Ng, & Sarri, 2006; Kenney, Reinholtz, & Angelini, 1997). Sexual abuse affects feelings about self and also judgments about what to expect in sexual relationships. Sexually abused children and teens have experienced a violation of their most private selves. This violation may contribute to feelings of powerlessness in relationships which may impair their ability to negotiate when to have sex and when to use condoms.

Sexual abuse contributes to earlier sexual initiation, more consensual sexual activity, more sexual partners, and an increased risk of sexual violence in intimate relationships (Taylor-Seehafer & Rew, 2000). Sexual abuse also increases risk for teen pregnancy and sexually transmitted and HIV infections as these youth are less likely to use condoms and contraception (Loeb et al., 2002). As discussed in Chapter 9, African American girls and women are at greater risk for sexual violence, including rape and date rape than girls in other ethnic groups.

Family Connection and Communication

Strong family bonding, communication, and parental monitoring protect girls from early and risky sexual activity. The findings from most studies show that adolescents who are connected to parents and family are more likely than those who do not have this connection to delay initiating sexual intercourse (McBride, Paikoff, & Holmbeck, 2003; Miller, 2002; Resnick et al., 1997). Dittus and Jaccard (2000) examined parental communication and sexual initiation using data from a national longitudinal study of over 10,000 teens. They found that teens who reported being highly satisfied with their relationship with their parents were three times less likely to engage in sex than teens who had little satisfaction with their parental relationships. These teens also were more likely to use birth control if sex occurred and less likely to become pregnant.

Communication with parents is an important ingredient for good sexual decisions. Girls who communicate about sex topics such as pregnancy, sexually transmitted infections, and HIV engage in less sex than those who do not. However, sometimes daughters do not communicate with their parents. O'Sullivan and colleagues (2001) conducted a study on parental communication between urban African American and Latino mothers and their preteen and teen daughters. The authors found that many mothers did not discuss topics other than biological issues and negative consequences of sexual activity with their daughters. The communication that did occur was often moralistic. The moralistic tone had the effect of discouraging daughters from confiding in their mothers. Girls who receive moralistic and preaching messages may be more likely to become secretly involved in romantic relationships without their mother's knowledge than those who receive clear and factual messages about sexuality.

Ashcraft (2004)[1] interviewed African American mothers and daughters about what they talked about with regard to relationships and sex. Ashcraft was interested in examining both mother's and daughter's communication about sexual topics and relationships. Girls and their mothers resided within an urban low-income housing community. Fifteen mother and daughter pairs were interviewed. Girls were between the ages of 11–14. Ashcraft found that mothers tended to tell their daughters not to have boyfriends. One daughter said "She said if she found out I had boyfriends she'd wear me out. So I didn't let her find out" (p. 101). When mothers talked about sex they tended to discuss contraception and to not discuss intimacy and emotions within relationships.

Mothers in the study by Ashcraft reported that they discussed contraception with their daughters telling them it was a means for preventing pregnancy and disease. However, daughters did not remember having discussions about contraception with their mothers. The discussions that did occur tended to focus on pregnancy rather than disease prevention. However, some of the girls were told by their mothers to use condoms even if using other methods of birth control such as birth control pills and DepoProvera shots.

Ashcraft also found that there was a lack of discussion regarding intimacy and emotions within relationships. She noted that the low level of discussion regarding emotions and intimacy is important because many of the girls she interviewed tended to equate love with receiving money or material things. Several of the girls in this study felt that the way you know that a boy or man cares for you is when he

---

[1] This was a doctoral dissertation study supervised by the author.

brings you presents. Such thinking can lead to poor decisions about engaging in sex especially if the teen feels that one way to reciprocate love is through sex. Not all girls felt that a good relationship involved money and material things. Some of the girls reported that trust, support, and care should be present in a relationship.

Jaccard, Dittus, and Gordon (1998) found a lack of congruency in youth and mother report of communication about their children's sexual behavior. Seven-hundred-forty-five African American youth aged 14–17 and their parents participated in this study. They found that mothers underestimated the extent to which their children were engaged in sexual activity. For example, 58% of teens in their sample reported sexual activity, but 34% of the mothers reported that their child had engaged in sexual activity. Mothers who underestimated their child's sexual activity tended to be those who did not talk to their child about sex. Also, teens tended to underestimate the extent to which they believed their mothers disapproved of them engaging in sex. Teens who underestimated mothers' disapproval of sex also tended to talk less with their mothers about sex. Ashcraft found similar findings regarding sexual activity in her interviews with mothers and daughters. She found that mothers did not know that their daughters were sexually active and that they reported having more conversations about sex than their daughter remembered.

Family factors are instrumental in the age of sexual debut. McBride, Paikoff, & Holmbeck (2003) interviewed 198 African American fourth and fifth graders and their families at Time 1 and two and a half years later at Time 2. The sample was recruited from an urban area. Data were collected on demographic variables and family conflict. At Time 2, 33.3% of the boys and 11.7% of the girls reported sexual initiation. Family conflict was associated with sexual initiation. Teens, who perceived greater conflict in the family, were more likely to report sexually debut. The level of pubertal development was also a factor in this relationship. The association between perceived family conflict and sexual initiation was greater for those youth at more advanced stages of pubertal development. The authors speculate that parents' perception of children's transition to adult status may have led to some restrictions which may have increased parental conflict.

In overview, a lack of family communication especially regarding sexual activity along with family conflict is likely to lead to more and earlier sexual activity. The father also has an impact on his daughter's sexual behavior as discussed next.

Father's Influence on Daughter's Sexual Behavior

Fathers influence their daughter's sexual behaviors (Rink, Tricker, & Harvey, 2007). One of the more long-term studies of the impact of fathers was carried out in the United States ($n = 242$) and New Zealand ($n = 530$) (Ellis et al., 2003). A longitudinal design allowed researchers to follow girls from age 5 to 18. The study found that girls in a father-absent household, especially households where fathers were absent for the first 5 years of their lives had more early sexual activity and teen pregnancy than girls raised in households with fathers present during their earlier years. Interestingly, the authors noted that father absence had a stronger effect on teen sexuality and pregnancy than other outcomes such as academic achievement and mental health. While this study was not specific to African American girls, the findings strongly point to father influence on sexual behaviors and consequences.

Research conducted with African American girls indicates that they are less likely to engage in sex if they believe that their father disapproves of them being sexually active. Dittus, Gordon, and Jaccard (1997) examined how daughter's perception of her father's attitude toward premarital sexual intercourse affected her sexual behavior. Data were collected from approximately 750 African American youth who resided within an inner city. The researchers found that girls' perceptions of father's attitudes were predictive of their sexual behavior. This effect occurred regardless of the perception of the teen's mother.

In overview, there has been limited literature and research on African American fathers with regard to their daughter's sexual behavior. What we can glean from the data that are available is that father involvement, communication, and relationships are important. Influences outside the family also impact sexual behavior.

Media Messages

The media has a pervasive and powerful influence on teen sexual behavior. Teens obtain information about sex and contraception from the media and the media provides role models of how to behave in sexual situations. A survey by The Kaiser Family Foundation (2001) indicated that 65% of 15- to 17-year-olds reported that they got information about birth control from advertising, 58% from television, 58% from magazine articles, and 39% from the Internet.

Media messages about sexuality are mixed. Some messages encourage girls to remain abstinent while at the same time she is surrounded by images of sexually attractive people behaving sexually often while drinking. These images also show young, single people engaging in casual sex with no contraception being discussed or used. Nor do the media typically show the consequences of unprotected sex, including sexually transmitted infections and pregnancy.

Television is a prime source for sexual information since it is readily accessible. In an analysis of prime time television, researchers found that the average adolescent in the United States views 14,000 sexual references, jokes, and innuendos each year. (Strasburger, 1997). Teens who watch 3–5 hour of TV each day witness about 2,000 sex acts per year. This includes kissing, embracing, implied intercourse, and fondling (Roberts, Foehr, Rideout, & Brodie, 1996). African American children and adolescents watch more television than other Americans and spend about 5 hour a day watching television (Ward, 2004).

In fact, the amount of time a teen spends watching television has been found to be a predictor of sexual activity. In one study, watching sex on television predicted who was involved in sexual activity and may have sped up the beginning of sexual activity. Collins et al. (2004) found a significant correlation between the amount of sexual content viewed by teens and advances in their sexual behavior during the subsequent year. They speculate that the reason for this increase is that young teens began to emulate the sexual behavior of older teens they see on television.

The media indirectly impact sexual behaviors among African American girls and women in other ways. Derogatory stereotypes may be internalized with resulting damage to self-worth and low expectations for good sexual and relationship choices (Stephens & Phillips, 2004).

Drug Use

Drug use is often a precursor to sexual activity. Although African American adolescent girls consume fewer drugs than girls from other ethnic groups, this is changing and drug use among African American girls has increased. The Center for Disease Control reports that among all sexually active students, 23.3% had drunk alcohol or used drugs before their last sexual intercourse. White (25.0%) and Hispanic (25.6%) students were more likely to drink alcohol and use drugs before sex than African American (14.1%) students. White female (20.5%) and Hispanic female (18.7%) students consumed more alcohol and drugs that did than African American female (12.8%) students. Also White male (29.9%) and Hispanic male (32.2%) students used more alcohol and drugs prior to sex than did African American males (15.4%). In general, these statistics suggest that sex is not paired with drug use among African American girls to the degree that it is with girls from other ethnic groups.

Marijuana is consumed in similar amounts by African American youth and youth from other ethnic groups. According to the CDC (2008), the prevalence of ever having smoked marijuana was slightly higher for African American students (39.6%) than White (38%) and Hispanic (38.9%) students. The prevalence of ever having smoked marijuana was also slightly higher for African American females (35%) than White females (34.1%) but slightly lower than for Hispanic female (35.9%) students. Marijuana lowers inhibition and impairs judgment regarding sexual decisions. Drug use among African American girls is discussed in more detail in Chapter 7.

Girls often initiate drug use within a family or romantic relationship. Drug use initiation may begin in the home with older siblings, cousins, and sometimes adult family members. Older male boyfriends also introduce girls to alcohol and drugs. Older partners have access to drugs and the resources to purchase drugs.

Teen Pregnancy, Births, and Parenting

Consequences of sexual activity include pregnancy, births, and parenting. These are discussed next.

Pregnancy

In 2002, the overall teenage pregnancy rate was estimated at 76.4 pregnancies per 1,000 females aged 15–19 years, down 10% from 2000 (84.8 per 1,000), and 35% lower than in 1990 (116.8 per 1,000) (Ventura, Abma, Mosher, & Henshaw, 2006). Despite this decline, the U.S. teenage pregnancy rate is still among the highest industrialized nations. Pregnancies among African American girls have had the highest rate of decline but still occur at higher rates than among girls in other racial and ethnic group. Among African American girls, pregnancy rates were 5.9/1,000 among girls under the age of 15, and 100.7/1,000 among girls between the ages of 15 and 17. Pregnancy rates for White girls under the age of 15 were 0.8/1,000, and 32.5/1,000 among girls aged 15–17. Latina pregnancy rates were 3.0/1,000 among girls under 15 and 83.1/1,000 for girls aged 15–17. Given the rates of teen pregnancy among African American adolescent females, there is clearly a need for more prevention programs specifically targeting pregnancy reduction. Risk and protective factors for teen pregnancy are similar to factors for teen parenting and will be discussed later.

Teen Births and Parenting

After a decline in teen birth rates from 1991 to 2006, birth rates increased for the first time in 15 years (Hamilton, Martin, & Ventura, 2007). The birth rate for U.S. teenagers 15–19 years increased by 3% to 41.9 births per 1,000 females in 2006. However, the birth rate of young teens 10–14 did not increase and this rate is 0.6/1,000. The birth rate for African American teens increased by 5% to 63.7/1,000 births. The rate increased by 2% for Latina teens to 83/1,000; there was a 2% increase for White teens to 26.6/1,000. The rate for Asian Pacific Island teen remained unchanged at 16.7/1,000. About one-fourth of the births to teens aged 15–19 are to African American girls; African American teen girls comprise 16% of the teen population (Centers for Disease Control, 2008).

Teen parenting can be challenging for the girl and her family. Many teen parents continue their education, complete high school, and even go on to attend college. However, education and other life-course expectations are generally compromised. An advocate for a youth group published the following statistics on what happens when girls become teen parents.

    http://www.advocatesforyouth.org/PUBLICATIONS/factsheet/fsadlchd.htm

1. Teen parenting reduces the level of education by 1–3 years.
2. African American and Hispanic teens who do not have children until age 20 or older are three to five times more likely to attend college than those who become parents before the age of 20.
3. Becoming a parent at an early age negatively affects employment opportunities and marital choices.

4. Teen mothers are more likely to be poor. About 25% of teen mothers live below the poverty level.
5. There is an intergenerational pattern of teen parenting among African Americans. The children of teen mothers are more likely to become teen parents themselves.
6. When African American girls become teen parents, their education is less affected than White or Hispanic girls.

This last point bears some discussion. When African American teens become parents, they are not as likely to stop their education as girls from other racial and ethnic groups. Girls who become parents often receive support from family members, most often their mother and grandmother but also siblings, aunts, and others in the immediate and extended family. Care and responsibility for the child is often shared among all family members.

What Contributes to Teen Pregnancies and Parenthood?

Several factors contribute to teen pregnancy and parenthood. Also, while some teen pregnancies are unplanned, some are not.

Pleasing Boyfriend

Some girls become pregnant because they think this is what will please their boyfriend. Boyfriends, especially older males, may pressure girls to have a child believing that this will tie her closer to him. Having a child may be seen as a sign of love and long-term commitment to a relationship. Similarly, some girls become pregnant because of the fear of losing her boyfriend and the belief that a child will make her partner less likely to leave her.

Davies and colleagues (2003) studied this issue. The researchers interviewed 462 sexually active African American teen girls between 14 and 18 years old who lived in low-income neighborhoods. Forty percent of the participants had a previous pregnancy. The researchers found that teens who thought that their boyfriends wanted a baby were 12 times more likely to wish they were pregnant than those who did not think their boyfriend wanted a baby. Moreover, those girls who became pregnant were almost four times as likely to have a partner who was at least 5 years older than they were. The researchers note that these girls may have believed that their boyfriends held the power in their sexual relationships. Also, the fact that their partners were older and perceived to not want to use condoms may have resulted in girls wanting to get pregnant and to have their boyfriends' baby. The researchers recommended that when there are older male–younger female relationships, the older male along with the younger female should be targeted in teen pregnancy prevention efforts.

Desire to Have Children

Some teen girls want to get pregnant. In the same study by Davis and colleagues, girls were asked whether they wanted to become pregnant. The researchers found that 24% expressed some desire to become pregnant in the near future. A baby may represent love, attention from family members, being perceived as grown, and as noted previously, a commitment to the relationship with the child's father.

Communities Influence Who Becomes a Parent

Girls who live in poor neighborhoods with fewer resources, employment, and positive adult role models tend to engage in more risky sexual activity than those who do live in these types of neighborhoods. Girls in these communities may see teen parenting as normative. Some researchers have speculated that early parenting occurs in those communities where girls may not have other opportunities (i.e., employment, education) to symbolize their transition from adolescence to adulthood. Parenting provides such a symbol of transition to adulthood.

South and Baumer (2000) used data from the National Survey of Children to examine the effects of community and race on adolescent premarital childbearing. A significant finding from this study was that the higher rates of adolescent childbearing among African American teens compared to White teens can be attributed to differences in the types of neighborhoods these two groups live in. African American teens are more likely than White teens to live in economically disadvantaged communities, and this is a primary reason for higher rates of childbearing. The study also found that teens in economically disadvantaged communities (compared to economically advantaged communities) have peers who believe that teenage premarital childbearing is normative.

There are several factors that protect African American girls from early and risk sexual behaviors. These factors, discussed in earlier chapters, include strong ethnic identity, religiosity, good family communication and cohesion, and community assets.

Health Consequences of Early Sexual Activity

Early and unprotected sexual activity brings with it many negative consequences, including sexually transmitted infections and HIV.

HIV and Sexually Transmitted Infections

HIV infection and AIDS is one of the most challenging problems currently facing the African American community. African American female adolescents account for 66% of AIDS cases among adolescents even though they comprise only 15% of the U.S. adolescent population (CDC, 2004). In comparison, White teens comprised 11% of AIDS cases and accounted for 63% of the teenage population. Sexual intercourse is the primary way in which African American adolescent females become infected. African American girls are more likely to begin sexual activity at a younger age and to have more partners. Her partners are also older. Girls may see older partners as more responsible and reliable than younger partners and not worry about using condoms.

However, older partners put girls at risk as they have had more sexual partners themselves, they are likely to have concurrent sexual partners, and/or to be infected with sexually transmitted diseases (Begley, Crosby, DiClemente et al., 2003). Older partners also have more power in the relationship and greater influence over sexual decisions than younger partners. Younger females are more likely to be persuaded by older partners and less likely to negotiate condom use.

Other Risk Factors for HIV

Girls are also at increased risk for HIV and sexually transmitted infections if a male partner injects drugs or has sex with other men. Men on the down low may feel safer with a younger female partner because he may feel that she has less power in the relationship and would be less likely than an older sexual partner to question his whereabouts and his activities. A younger partner is also less likely to recognize deception and behavior that provide clues to down-low behavior. The risk factors of partner injection drug use and being on the down low do not result in any greater risk for African American teens than for females from other racial and ethnic groups (CDC, HIV/AIDS Surveillance Report 2005).

Why do African American Girls Have the Highest Risk for HIV?

The majority of African American teens use condoms during sexual intercourse. In fact, the rate of condom use among African American teens is slightly higher than that of youth in other racial and ethnic groups. So why are HIV and prevalence rates higher among African American teens (and adults)? The answer lies in the fact that the overall prevalence of HIV is higher, so more sexual partners are infected. Health care disparities, including access to preventive messages and programs, contribute to this increase in HIV infection rates.

Summary

Sexuality is an important aspect of a girl's identity and her sexual decisions affect her life in several ways. Overall African American girls have higher rates of sexual activity than girls from other ethnic groups. Condom use is slightly higher among African American girls than girls from other ethnic groups. Several factors contribute to teen sexual activity, including puberty, self-esteem, family communication, the media, and the community in which she resides. Sexual abuse is also a major contributor to early and risky sexual activity.

Teen pregnancy and birth rates declined for years but recently showed an increase and remain the highest of any industrial Western nation. The consequences of teen parenting can be adverse although African American girls tend to complete their schooling when they become parents. Girls need to understand the consequences of early and risky sex and be given the skills to refuse sexual activity. The strength she possesses within herself along with support from her family and community can shield her during this period.

Recommendation and Resources

Provide Accurate Sexual Information

Teens need accurate information about sexuality, accessible access to resources, and the skills and beliefs to resist engaging in early and unprotected sex. Education should include accurate information on physical development, contraception, and abstinence. Within discussions of education, teens should be provided with the opportunity to explore their values, relationships, gender role beliefs, sexual orientation, and sexual decision making. There is an abundance of information available on the web and there are several books and articles that have been published. Some books have been written by teens themselves. Some of these resources are listed under the resource section. However, we know that education is not sufficient by itself to change behavior. Several research-based curriculums have been developed and evaluated and found effective in reducing early and risky sexual activity and associated risks.

Reduce Sexual Behavior and Risk

Several researchers have implemented and evaluated programs that show good results for reducing sexual risk, teen pregnancies, and HIV and sexually transmitted infections among African American girls. These curricula can be carried out in schools, community centers, health clinics, churches, and other organizations.

Becoming a Responsible Teen

Becoming a Responsible Teen (B.A.R.T.) is an HIV prevention curriculum for African American adolescents, aged 14–18. B.A.R.T. was developed by Dr. St. Lawrence and colleagues (1995) and is carried out in community settings. This curriculum designed for single-sex groups, consists of eight sessions, which lasts for about 2 hour each. It includes group discussions and role play activities. The role play activities were developed by teens. In this program, teens learn to "spread the word" to their friends about HIV risks. They practice skills learned within the group in situations in the real world.

Although the primary goal of B.A.R.T is HIV prevention, the curriculum also includes topics and activities on teen pregnancy prevention. Teens discuss their values about sexual decisions and pressures as well as practice skills to reduce sexual risk taking. They learn correct condom use, assertive communication, refusal techniques, self-management, and problem solving. Abstinence is also discussed throughout the curriculum.

Individuals can receive training and further information, including costs from: ETR Associates Phone: 1-800-321-4407; Fax: 1-800-435-8433; Internet: www.etr.org.

Be Proud! Be Responsible! A Safer Sex Curriculum

This curriculum also addresses HIV and sexually transmitted infection prevention by improving HIV-related knowledge, attitudes, and behaviors (Jemmott, Jemmott, & Fong 1992) among teens aged 13–18. There are six sessions that lasts for 50 minutes. The program has been used with African American youth especially those who reside in urban and inner-city communities. This program addresses the importance of protecting one's community, as well as oneself against the potentially negative consequences of unprotected sexual intercourse. The curriculum covers topics such as self-esteem and self-respect by emphasizing that it feels good to make proud and responsible safer sex decisions.

For further information contact select Media: Phone, 1.800.707.6334; Web, http://www.selectmedia.org. For educator training, contact ETR Associates: Phone, 1.800.321.4407; Fax, 1.800.435.8433; Web, http://www.etr.org.

Making Proud Choices! was developed by the same researchers as the Be Proud! Be Responsible! Curriculum for younger African American teens aged 11–13. This HIV prevention curriculum emphasizes safer sex, including information about abstinence and condoms. Making Proud Choices! has eight sessions, each lasting 60 minutes. It includes experiential activities to build skills to delay initiating sex and to communicate with partners. It also teaches sexually active youth to use condoms.

For More Information or to Order, Contact Select Media: Phone, 1.800.707.6334; Web, http://www.selectmedia.org. For information regarding training, contact ETR: Phone, 1.800.321.4407; Fax, 1.800.435.8433.

Increasing Media Literacy Regarding Sexual Activity

Given that the media contributes to sexual behavior, a way to promote sexual responsibility is to use the media in prevention efforts. Media literacy provides adolescents with the skills needed to access, analyze, and evaluate communicate messages in a variety of forms (Hobbs, 1997). Media literacy has been implemented in community centers and schools across the nation. Youth and parents are taught to be critical media consumers by showing them how media messages are constructed. By deconstructing these messages, teens can uncover their assumptions and hidden values and the subtle influence these messages have (Thoman, 1998). A comprehensive interactive web-based media literacy program designed for teens and adults is listed under the resources.

Evaluate Sexual Messages

Convene students in small groups of about four to five persons. Let each group represent movies and TV shows, commercials, magazine articles, print ads, or music lyrics. Have each group develop a checklist for evaluating sexual messages. Discuss the characters, their clothing, and their verbal and nonverbal communication. Have the teens identify what sexual messages are implicit and what sexual messages are subtle.

Provide Contraceptive Services

Teens should have access to accessible and affordable contraceptive services. Comprehensive sexual and reproductive health services for teens should include gynecological exams, discussion of contraceptive methods, pregnancy testing, and screening, treatment, and/or referral for sexually transmitted infections. There is varied opinion as to whether these services should be provided without parental knowledge and consent and each individual/agency will have to make this determination considering local policies. Males should also be involved in family planning efforts and teens should bring along their male partners. Contraceptive services should be offered during accessible hours, including walk-in appointments, and flexible and extended hours during evenings and weekends. They should be available in convenient settings where teens gather. Services should be free of charge or on a sliding fee. The following website provides lots on information on contraceptive services for youth. http://www.advocatesforyouth.org/publications/iag/component.htm

Encourage Abstinence Through Virginity Clubs

Virginity clubs have become common in some schools and communities. Originally implemented within religious institutions, they have become common in nonreligious institutions and are now in many high schools, including predominately African American schools. Participants in Virginity clubs make a pledge to remain abstinent until marriage.

Research is mixed regarding the effectiveness of abstinence in preventing sexual activity and related outcomes. Some studies have shown no benefit of abstinence only programs, while other programs continue to be implemented. It is likely that these programs may be useful for individuals who have religious and moral beliefs that abstinence is the right choice for them.

Reduce Sexual Activity and Risk Through Small Group and Classroom Activities

Interview Teen Parents

Have students' interview adults who were and were not teen parents about their adolescence. They can ask the adult how they prepared for adulthood. Students should prepare a list of questions to ask prior to the interview. These interviews can be videotaped and or summarized by teens in an edited book.

Invite a panel of teen mothers and fathers to discuss their parenthood experience, including the pros and cons, sacrifices and benefits, and so on. Have questions prepared prior to the panel discussion.

Have Girls Practice Sexual Refusal

Working in small groups, ask students to develop specific refusal responses to the following sexual pressure statements: "Everybody's doing it, why not you? If you won't, I guess this is the end for us. You would if you cared for me." Students can role play their responses.

Write Essays on Topics Related to Sexual Decisions

Have teens write short essays on topics such as: (a) Why wait until marriage; (b) How peer pressure affects sex decision; (c) How parents influence sexual decisions; (d) How does feelings about yourself affect sexual decisions; (e) When is a good time to began dating?

Resources

Teen Source. This is a sex education resource about sexual health and relationship for teens written by teens. (www.teensource.org)

Sex education: Talking to your teen about sex. Resource for parents to help them to communicate with their daughter. http://www.cnn.com/HEALTH/library/sex-education/CC00032.html

Talking About Sex with Teens Family Education. This website provides information for parents on how to talk to teens. (http://life.familyeducation.com/sex/teen/34505.html)

Teen Aware, Sex, Media, and You. This is an interactive comprehensive web site that uses media literacy as a strategy for abstinence-based sex education. It provides several modules that can be used by adults working with teens and can also be used by teens themselves. (http://depts.washington.edu/taware)

Chapter 9
Prosocial Behavior and Aggression

> *"I believe in God. I believe that if it wasn't for Him, we*
> *wouldn't be here. I wouldn't have the talents that I have. I can*
> *sing, I can dance, poetry ... my favorite poet is Maya Angelou*
> *and Langston Hughes, and I just like me being here. That's my*
> *belief in God."*
>
> *A teen girl in a focus group who responded to question,*
> *"what are your beliefs in God (or a higher power)?"*

African American girls engage in both positive and hurtful behaviors, and these behaviors are the topics of this chapter. Prosocial behaviors include showing care and concern, altruistic acts, and cooperation. Morality, religiosity, and spirituality are often linked to prosocial behaviors, and these are also discussed in this chapter. The quote above is an example of one girl's feelings about God. Aggressive behaviors are counter to prosocial behaviors and include aggression, bullying, and violence as well as relational aggression, a type of aggression that may be more unique to females. Girls are often the victims of acts of violence, including date rape.

This chapter examines the causes and consequences of prosocial and aggressive behavior. The chapter begins with a discussion of prosocial behavior, then religion and spirituality. Aggression, violence, and sexual victimization are also discussed. The chapter concludes with "Recommendations and Resources" for increasing prosocial behavior and decreasing aggression by and against girls.

Prosocial Behaviors

Prosocial behavior includes behaviors such as sharing, helping, and cooperating. Prosocial behavior among adolescents is associated with social competence, high self-esteem, emotional strength, and positive and fulfilling interpersonal

F.Z. Belgrave, *African American Girls*, Advancing Responsible Adolescent Development, 141
DOI 10.1007/978-1-4419-0090-6_9, © Springer Science+Business Media, LLC 2009

relationships (Wentzel, Filisetti, & Looney, 2007). While there has been a fair amount written on aggression and other antisocial behaviors among adolescents, less has been written on prosocial behavior. Even less has been written on prosocial behaviors among African American girls.

Wentzel and colleagues developed a model of adolescent prosocial behavior that helps us understand who and under what conditions prosocial behavior is enacted. Prosocial behavior is determined by one's personal goal to engage in prosocial behavior. Personal goals are influenced by self-processes such as empathy, affect, perspective taking, and perceived competence. The model also includes perceived expectations for prosocial behavior – what are the expectations from those in the youth's environment regarding prosocial behavior. Wentzel and colleagues tested this model by examining peer and teacher reports of prosocial behavior, self-processes, and expectations among 339 sixth and eighth graders. Fifty-two percent of the sample comprised girls and 44% was African American. Prosocial behavior was defined as helping and sharing as reported by the students' peers and teachers. The authors found some gender and ethnic differences in how these three factors affected prosocial behavior. Peers and teachers reported that girls (compared to boys) engaged in more prosocial behavior, and girls also reported higher levels of empathy and perceived that their teachers and peers expected them to behavior in prosocial ways.

Among White students perceived expectations from peers were correlated with prosocial behavior. If students believed that peers expected prosocial behavior they were more likely to display prosocial behaviors. However, perceived expectations from peers were not correlated with prosocial behavior among African American students. The authors speculated that this might be due to the fact that African Americans were not the racial majority in this school setting. Expectations from peers for prosocial behavior might contribute to prosocial behavior if African American students are in schools in which they are the racial majority and not the racial minority. Also, as discussed in Chapter 4, African American adolescent behavior may be less influenced by peers than other ethnic groups. This might account for the insignificant correlations between peer expectation and prosocial behavior among African American students. Clearly, more research is needed on models of and determinants of prosocial behavior among African American adolescents, including African American girls.

Although there has been limited literature on this topic, one might expect relational and communal beliefs and values found among females and people of African descent to contribute positively to prosocial behavior. Relational values imply that the self is influenced by others and cooperation and concern for others would follow from this (Miller, 1991). Also, Africentric communal values of caring for and feeling responsible for those within one's social groups should affect the extent to which prosocial behavior is enacted (Belgrave & Allison, 2006).

Prosocial Behavior Among African American Adolescents

A few studies have examined prosocial behaviors among African American adolescents. Esposito (2007)[1] examined prosocial behavior in a sample of 177 African American sixth-, seventh-, and eighth-grade middle school youth. Prosocial behaviors were assessed with questions that included whether the students tried to cheer up other kids who felt upset or sad, the students said or did nice things for other students, and whether they assisted others in need (Crick & Grotpeter, 1995).

Esposito found that 35% of the students reported frequently engaging in prosocial behaviors almost all the time or all the time. She found that girls were significantly more likely to engage in prosocial behavior than boys. These behaviors included assisting others in need, saying or doing nice things for peers, and cheering persons up with they were sad or upset. Empathy was also associated with prosocial behavior in this sample and is discussed next.

Empathy

Empathy is one factor that contributes to prosocial behavior. Empathy is an emotional response that comes from feeling the emotional state of another individual (Feshbach, 1997). Empathy also involves the ability to take on the perspective of another. Girls tend to report higher levels of empathy than boys. In this study, Esposito found that girls reported higher levels of empathy than boys. Also, empathy was correlated with prosocial behaviors for girls more so than for boys.

An adolescent's ability to engage in perspective taking is an important requirement for empathy and prosocial behavior. Perspective taking can be taught in skill development programs and is one way in which prosocial behavior can be increased (see "Recommendation and Resource" section).

McMahon, Wernsman, and Parnes (2006) studied the relationship between empathy and prosocial behavior in a sample of African American youth in early adolescence. They also looked at whether this relationship differed for boys and girls. Similar to the findings in the Esposito study, the authors found that empathy was associated with prosocial behaviors. Also, while the relationship between empathy and prosocial behavior was significant for both males and females, it was more pronounced for males. This finding differed from the one in the Esposito study where the relationship between empathy and prosocial behavior was more pronounced for females than males. A construct related to prosocial behavior is morality and is discussed next.

---

[1] Esposito's research was a doctoral dissertation supervised by the author.

Morality

Moral reasoning considers how individuals conform themselves to function in society and considers concepts such as fairness, justice, and consideration for others. Hence, morality may be viewed as a type of prosocial attitude and value. Woods and Jagers (2003) describe components of morality and cultural values related to morality in a sample of African American adolescents. Components of morality discussed by Woods and Jagers include (1) affect and care; (2) communal values; and (3) spirituality. Woods and Jagers noted that cultural values are inherent to understanding morality. Affect and care are identified as sensitivity and receptivity to the emotional cues of others, and these are associated with higher levels of moral reasoning. According to Woods and Jagers, girls have a morality of care that is based on connections with others, while boys may develop a morality of justice based on fairness. They note that communal values found among African Americans support the development of morality of care. A second component of morality is communalism which reflects the African belief in collective identity and the extended self. Accordingly, a high value is placed on social relationships and the good of the group should take priority over the needs of the individual (Turiel & Neff, 2000). A third component of morality is spirituality and religion (these will be discussed in the next section).

Woods and Jagers administered measures of communalism, affect, spirituality, and moral reasoning to 50 African American eighth-grade students. They found that the values of communalism, spirituality, and affect were significantly associated with moral reasoning for both girls and boys. They authors also found that female adolescents reported higher levels of affect than did males. Altruistic behavior is a type of prosocial behavior and is discussed next.

Altruistic Behavior

Altruism is demonstrated by a concern for the welfare of others without expectation of anything in return. In an interesting study of altruistic behavior in a sample of African American and Latina adolescents, Hart and Fegley (1995) identified adolescents who had demonstrated exemplary behaviors in caring for others. Calling these adolescents care exemplars, Hart and Fegley noted that the accomplishments of these individuals were remarkable given that they were from economically distressed communities. The authors were interested in how adolescents who had demonstrated exemplary care for others conceptualized self.

Care exemplars included adolescents who had (1) been involved in community, church, or youth groups that benefited others; (2) unusual and commendable family responsibilities; and (3) volunteered time to help others. Fifteen adolescents nominated as care exemplars by members of the community were included in the final interview sample. Once these individuals were identified, they were matched with adolescents of the same age, gender, ethnicity, and from the same neighborhood for comparison purposes. The authors found that care exemplars had a different self-conceptualization than noncare exemplars. Care exemplars were more likely to describe themselves by mentioning moral personality traits and moral goals than comparison adolescents who were not care exemplars. In contrast to comparison adolescents, care exemplars were also more likely to say that their actual selves were consistent with their ideal selves and to identify with their parents. On the other hand, comparison adolescents were more likely to have actual selves that incorporated the self with respect to best friends. The authors noted that these differences suggested that care exemplars more so than comparison participants were more likely to be oriented toward their ideals and parental values. They noted that comparison adolescents had values more like suburban adolescents in which peers are more important than parents. This study did not specifically address differences in behaviors among males and females but does present an interesting analysis of how the self is conceptualized by African American and Latino youth who have demonstrated care for others. Can certain types of education influence prosocial values? This topic is discussed next.

Africentric Education

Certain educational and contextual factors can increase prosocial behavior. One study examined the impact of Africentric education on prosocial behavior. Pilgrim (2006) investigated whether students who participated in an Africentric educational program (e.g., a cooperative classroom climate, exposure to African American history/values and inclusion of family/community values) increased in prosocial behavior. Pilgrim recruited 184 African American fifth and sixth grade students from a predominately African American school. Pilgrim found that students who were in the Africentric education class rated themselves as engaging in more prosocial behavior than those not in the class.

In summary, goals and processes such as empathy and perspective taking affect whether an adolescent engages in prosocial behavior. African American girls are more likely to engage in prosocial behavior than boys and are more likely to have higher levels of empathy. Communal and relational values and connection to others are other determinants of prosocial behavior among African American adolescent girls. Adolescents who engage in exemplary prosocial behavior are likely to view themselves using moral descriptors and also see themselves as similar to parents. Spiritual and religious beliefs and practices affect prosocial behavior, and these are discussed next.

Spirituality and Religiosity

Spirituality and religiosity are generally linked to prosocial behavior although not exclusively. Adolescents vary greatly in spirituality and religiosity. Although the terms "spirituality" and "religiosity" are sometimes used interchangeably, they differ in meaning. Spirituality is a worldview that is central to cultural expressions found in the African Diaspora (Jagers & Smith, 1996). Spirituality is an individual's search for the state of transcendence, peace, connectedness, hope, purpose, and meaning in life that is often obtained through religious beliefs (McCormick, Holder, Wetsel, & Cawthon, 2001). On the other hand, religiosity is more focused on organized religion, which is an organized system of beliefs, practices, and rituals designed to enhance one's relationship with God (Taylor, Chatters, & Levin, 2004).

Smith, Denton, Faris, and Regnerus (2002) analyzed high school students' religious practices using data from several national data sources. They found that among 8th, 10th, and 12th graders, about 38% attend religious services weekly, 16% attend one to two times a month, 31% attend rarely, and 15% never attend religious services. About half of American adolescents participate in religious youth groups (Smith et al., 2000), and there are gender differences in participation. Twenty-eight percent of 12th grade girls, compared to 22% of 12th grade boys, have been involved in a religious youth group for the full 4 years of high school.

Religious service attendance among high school youth varies by racial/ethnic group. African American adolescents have the highest rates of church attendance, followed by Whites. African American high school students are also slightly more likely than White students to be involved in a religious youth group for all of their 4 years of high school. This rate is nearly twice the rate for youth from "other" racial and ethnic groups. Given higher attendance and participation in religious activities by African Americans and girls, we would expect African American girls to be especially involved in religious activities such as youth groups and attending worship services.

Being religious can be both intrinsic (more akin to spiritual beliefs) and extrinsic (religious practices). Milevsky and Levitt (2004) examined the impact of both extrinsic and intrinsic religiosity on psychological adjustment among 694 African American, White, and Latino students. The authors found that intrinsically religious adolescents scored more favorably with respect to psychological adjustment than those who were less intrinsically religious. Females and African Americans also scored higher on intrinsic religiosity. This finding also suggests that African American adolescent females are likely to have intrinsic religious beliefs.

Ball, Armistead, and Austin (2003) examined religiosity among a sample of 492 African American female adolescents aged 12–19. The study found that the vast majority of the adolescents reported a belief in God and attended religious services. The majority reported their religious faith as Christianity. The authors found that higher levels of religiosity were correlated with higher levels of self-esteem and overall better psychological functioning.

In overview, we expect African American girls to have both intrinsic and extrinsic religious beliefs and practices, and these beliefs and practices are linked to better psychological functioning. We next turn to the opposite of prosocial behavior and focus on aggression, including aggression toward girls.

Aggression and Violence

We turn our attention to behavior that is counter to prosocial behavior. Aggression is the intent to cause harm to others (Archer, 2001). Some of the causes of aggression and violence among African American girls are the same as for boys and youth in other racial and ethnic groups. Several family, personal, and community-level factors contribute to violence and aggression. For example, low family cohesion and support, parents' use of harsh physical discipline and punishment are associated with more aggressive behavior among youth (Baldry & Farrington, 2000; Shields & Cicchetti, 2001). Affiliating with peers who are delinquent and aggressive increases youth aggression and violence (Espelage, Bosworth, & Simon, 2000). Neighborhood factors such as crime, access to guns, drugs, and other environmental stressors also contribute to aggression and violence among youth. Youth living in urban neighborhoods are more likely to report seeing violence and being victims of violence than those who do not live in urban neighborhoods (Espelage, Bosworth, & Simon, 2000). Poverty is also associated with violence (Thomas & Bierman, 2006).

The study Esposito (2007) conducted on prosocial behavior also examined one type of aggression, bullying behavior among African American middle school students attending an urban school. Bullying occurs when a student is exposed repeatedly to negative behaviors on the part of one or more other students. When bullying occurs, there is generally an imbalance in strength between the bully and the victim, and the victim is usually unsuccessful at defending him/herself against the attack (Olweus, 1993).

Esposito was interested in the prevalence of bullying among African American students in early adolescence and whether boys and girls differed in bullying. She was also interested in whether girls and boys engage in different types of bullying. Nationally, approximately 10–15% of middle school students are classified as bullies (Solberg & Olweus, 2003). In her study, Esposito found that 24% of the participants reported bullying behaviors such as hitting, shoving, threatening, yelling at and taunting peers. Forty-seven percent reported physical aggression some of the time. Contrary to expectations, there were no gender differences in bullying. Girls did not bully any less than boys. Esposito speculated that one reason for the higher reported bullying among students in this sample may be due to socialization and culturally influenced roles and beliefs about what it means to defend and stand up for oneself. That is, African American children who reside within low-resource communities (where this study was conducted) may learn that it is beneficial to bully rather than be bullied. Another reason why there were no differences between males and females may be because African American females are likely to be androgynous and possess both masculine and feminine traits (see Chapter 2). Perhaps these traits contributed to higher levels of bullying among African American girls than what we might see in a national sample. Finally, many of the youth in this sample resided in low-resource communities where there are higher rates of crime. These youth may have learned bullying as a self-protective mechanism against potential harm to them.

While the rate of bullying was higher than reported national rates in this sample of African American students, it is also important to note that a large percentage (35%) of the students engaged in prosocial behavior (discussed earlier).

Relational Aggression

Another type of aggression often associated with females is relational aggression. Esposito also examined relational aggression in the study just discussed. Relational aggression involves behaviors such as gossiping, withdrawing affection to get what you want, and socially excluding others (Crick, Bigbee, & Howes, 1996). In the Esposito study, 6% of the students engaged in relational aggression. Research suggests that boys are more likely to engage in physical aggression and girls are more likely to engage in relational aggression (Crick, Bigbee, & Howes, 1996). However, in the Esposito study, girls did not engage in relational aggression more so than boys. In fact in this study, boys were slightly more likely to engage in relational aggression.

The findings from the Esposito study suggest that African American girls might be more similar to African American boys in aggressive behavior than to girls from other ethnic and racial groups. Also, the level of bullying was higher than national levels. In considering the findings from this study, the context in which the study was carried out should be considered. Studies conducted on aggression among African American girls, who reside in better-resourced communities, might show different results. Violence among girls is discussed next.

Violence Among Girls

The Surgeon General report indicated that between 15% and 30% of girls have committed a violent act by the age of 17 (Department of Health and Human Services, 2001). The nature of violence and the type of violence perpetuated by girls differ than from boys. Girls are more likely than boys to be violent at home and/or school and to aggress against parents, siblings, and other girls (Molnar, Roberts, Browne, Gardener, & Buka, 2004).

Molnar and colleagues interviewed girls to understand how they perceived their aggression and to obtain their suggestions for ways to prevent violence by girls. Sixty-one urban adolescent females, between the ages of 11 and 17, who had engaged in a violent act over the past year (e.g., hit someone and police was involved, threw objects like rocks or bottles at people, hit someone at home, etc.) were interviewed. The authors also asked girls about prosocial behavior such as participating in sports teams, school clubs, and volunteer work. Forty-two percent of the girls were African American, 25% were Latina, 15% were White, and 18% were other. The neighborhoods where girls lived were diverse with about 25% coming from the poorest and most unsafe neighborhood in the City. Interviewees were asked for suggestions on how to prevent negative and aggressive behavior and how to promote positive and prosocial behavior.

There were six themes that girls identified for what girls could do to stay safe (Molnar et al.). These were as follows: (1) Stay at home. About 18% of girls reported that their neighborhoods were very dangerous and that they could be attacked and/or put in risky situations such as gang activity or using drugs. Therefore, the best plan was to stay at home or to be in supervised activities at all times. (2) Stay away from dangerous people. About one-third of the girls indicated that there were dangerous people (peers, adults, boyfriends) who could harm them or involve them in criminal behaviors. (3) Stay busy with after-school activities. About a third of the girls reported that after-school activities kept them safe. (4) Stay calm. Girls reported that a peaceful and calm attitude was helpful when faced with a potential fight. (5) Use escorts. Girls reported having family and friends accompany them to keep them safe when in danger of violence. (6) Fight to prevent future fights. About a third of the girls believed that fighting was an appropriate action in some situations. These girls felt that they had to fight for self-defense, and when they fought back the aggressors did not bother them again.

These girls also identified resources that helped them to keep safe. These resources included their mothers, other family members, and also friends. Older girls were especially helpful in giving advice about how to stay safe. Girls are more likely to be a victim of violence than a perpetrator of violence and this is discussed next.

Violence Against Girls

Sexual Victimization

Although sexual victimization can occur among males, it is much more likely to occur among females. Using data from the national 2005 Youth Risk Behavior Survey, Howard, Wang, and Yan (2007a) report that overall 8.01% of high school adolescents had a lifetime history of forced sexual intercourse. The prevalence for females was 10.3% and the prevalence for males was 4.8%. Moreover, Howard and colleagues report that it is likely that these reported prevalence rates are underestimations of the actual extent of sexual violence.

There are significantly higher rates of forced sex among African American adolescents and women (9.6%) as compared to White adolescents and women (6.9%) (Grunbaum et al., 2002). Adolescent girls also experience more sexual victimization than older women. One study explored the prevalence of different types of sexual victimization among a sample of 249 African American adolescents, aged 14–19 years (Cecil & Matson, 2006). The authors were also interested in whether different forms of sexual victimization were associated with poorer psychosocial adjustment. Girls who were attending adolescent health care clinics were recruited for the study. About a third of the adolescents reported being raped (32.1%); one-third reported sexual coercion (33.7%). A little over 10% (10.8) reported an attempted rape. Only about a fourth of the adolescents (23.4%) reported never having been victimized. This rate is much higher than has been reported previously. However, this sample of adolescent females was low income, and low-income females have reported more rapes than those with higher incomes. Also, these girls were recruited from a clinical setting. Girls recruited from schools and other types of community settings might report different rates of sexual violence.

In the Cecil & Matson study (2006), girls who have been raped reported lower levels of self-esteem and competence than girls who had not been raped. Levels of self-esteem, depression, and mastery were also lower for girls who had been raped compared to girls who had experienced other forms of sexual coercion. These findings suggest that the ways in which girls experience sexual victimization will affect their emotional functioning. Girls who have been raped may need to have different interventions than those who have had other forms of sexual victimization.

Osborne and Rhodes (2001) reported similar findings in an earlier study of 275 pregnant and parenting African American and Latino adolescents aged 11–17. These authors found that close to 18% of these girls reported sexual victimization, mostly forced sexual intercourse. Adolescents who had been victimized reported higher levels of stress, depression, and anxiety than those who had not.

Dating Violence

Dating violence and date rape are of enormous concern. Girls who are victimized by relationship violence are more likely to have other problems such as depression, and/or engage in other risky behaviors such as drinking and drug use (Howard, Wang, & Yan, 2007b). Once violence begins in a relationship, girls are more likely to accept it in subsequent relationships. Clearly, interventions are needed to prevent dating violence in the first place.

Howard and colleagues (2007b) analyzed data from the Youth Risk Behavior Survey. The survey asked students if a boyfriend or a girlfriend had hit, slapped, or physically hurt them on purpose. They found that about 10.3% of teen girls reported experiencing physical dating violence. The percentage who reported being victimized was similar for both males and females. However, females reported that they were more likely than males to suffer injury and were more vulnerable to violent sexual abuse than males. Also, the authors found that younger adolescents (i.e., those in ninth grade) were no less likely to have been victimized than older adolescents (i.e., those in 12th grade).

African American girls were 1.5 times more likely to report that they had experienced physical dating violence compared to their White peers. African American girls who reported more physical dating violence were more likely to have engaged in fighting themselves, to have engaged in sexual activity, and to report being sad or depressed (Howard et al., 2007b).

Research suggests that many African American girls will be victimized by dating partners. The period of early adolescence is a critical period for intervening prior to girls starting to date, and prevention programs must address dating violence among both males and females. Also, prevention efforts must consider environmental and personal factors that contribute to partner victimization and date rape. One environmental factor that can be controlled is what television programs are watched. The content of certain television programming has been noted as a contributor to the acceptance of date rape among males (Kaestle, Halpern, & Brown, 2007). Particularly, higher levels of exposure to televised music videos and prowrestling were found to be associated with rape acceptance among males but not females middle school students. Male middle school students who watched more music videos and prowrestling were less likely to agree with the statement "forcing a partner to have sex is never OK" than those who watched less televised music videos and wrestling.

Raiford, Wingood, and DiClemente (2007) conducted one of the few studies that specifically looked at dating violence over a 1-year period among an African American female adolescent sample. Date violence was defined as ever having verbal or physical abuse from a boyfriend. Five-hundred-twenty-two African American females aged 14–18 participated in the study. Participants were recruited from a variety of sources, including health clinics and school health classes.

At the beginning of the study, 28% reported a history of dating violence. These adolescents were not included in subsequent analysis as the authors wanted to determine what additional percentage experienced dating violence during the 1-year period. One year later, 12% reported dating violence. The study found that adolescents who experienced date violence were twice more likely to report less understanding of healthy relationships and almost twice as likely to have viewed X-rated movies. Prevention programs that focus on healthy relationships might be helpful in preventing date rape.

When the victim of a rape is an African American girl or woman, she may not be taken as seriously or seen as credible as when the victim is White. In one study, both White and African American college students read a scenario describing a date that ended with a forced sexual encounter where the victim was African American or White (Foley, Evancic, Karnik, & King, 1995). They found that forcible sexual encounter was seen as less serious when the victim was an African American woman than when the victim was a White woman.

Same-Sex Dating Violence

There has been very little research on same-sex dating violence. The scant research that exists suggests that dating violence occurs at similar rates to opposite partner violence. Data from adolescents who reported same-sex intimate relationships from the National Longitudinal Study of Adolescent Health were analyzed (Halpern, Young, Waller, Martin, & Kupper, 2004). More females (26%) report psychological violence than males (14.6%). Twenty-eight percent of females and 24% of males reported physical violence. Adolescents in same-sex relationships have the additional threat and fear of their partner outing them (Freedner, Freed, Yang, & Austin, 2002). No studies could be located on dating violence among same-sex African American adolescent girls.

Preventing Teen Dating Violence

Compared to boys, girls are more likely to be involved in more severe types of violence and to be raped. When African American women are raped, their credibility is less than that of White women. Programs to help youth see how the media contribute to violence against women may be helpful. These programs can involve parents and concerned others in discussions with their sons and daughters about violence against women. Programs at schools, churches, and communities that address partner violence and rape are also important.

Understanding what a healthy relationship looks like is another strategy. During early adolescence, dating and relationships are new experiences for girls. When they began a relationship for the first time, they may not even know what relationship violence is. Most adolescents would know that physical attacks such as hitting, slapping, and kicking are violent. However, emotional violence is an equally hurtful form of violence. Emotional violence includes being called names, humiliation, and threats. Girls need to know what is and is not acceptable in a relationship.

Parental modeling of abusive relationships is also detrimental to young girls understanding of a healthy relationship. In our discussions with and interviews with African American girls, many have told us that their mother, aunt, or sister was abused by or in an abusive relationship with a male partner (Ashcraft, 2004). Although these girls recognize the problems with abuse relationships, it does not always stop them from being in a similar relationship and repeating the cycle of abuse. There are several good internet sites that offer tips to stop teen dating violence, and these are provided in the section on "Recommendations and Resources."

In overview, African American girls and boys may not differ in types of aggressive behaviors as much as girls and boys from other ethnic groups. This may in part be due to more similar gender role socialization among African American boys and girls where both girls and boys are socialized to be androgynous. African American girls are likely to experience more sexual victimization, including more severe forms of sexual victimization such as rape and date rape when compared to girls from other ethnic groups.

Summary

Prosocial behaviors include showing care and concern, altruistic actions, and cooperation. Determinants of prosocial behavior include empathy and perspective taking, and expectations from others. Relational and communal values contribute to prosocial behavior among African American girls. Another factor related to proso-cial behavior is morality which has been linked to communal values and spirituality. Spiritual and religious beliefs also promote prosocial behavior and well-being. Spir-itual beliefs and religious practices are higher among girls than boys and among African Americans than other ethnic groups. African American girls are especially likely to possess spiritual and religious beliefs and practices.

Aggression is the intent to cause harm to another. Because of similar gender role beliefs and socialization practices among African American girls and boys, we see fewer differences in prosocial behavior, aggression, and relational aggression among African American females and males. This is in contrast to other racial and ethnic groups in which physical aggression is higher among males and relational aggression is higher among females.

Sexual victimization is of major concern for girls and women. Research has indi-cated high levels of sexual victimization among African American girls and women, and African American females are more likely to be victims of forced intercourse than women from other racial and ethnic groups. They are also more likely to be vic-tims of date rape. Intervention programs that focus on healthy relationships should help girls and boys to understand what healthy relationships are and decrease sexual victimization.

Reinforcing communal and relational values can support the development of African American adolescent girls' prosocial behavior. Spiritual and religious activ-ities are likely to further support her development in this area. Positive feelings about herself, family communication and cohesion, and healthy school and community environments are likely to deter her from destructive and abusive relationships.

Recommendations and Resources

Increasing Prosocial Behavior

Yael Kidron and Steve Fleischman (2006) provide three strategies that can be used to increase prosocial behavior in the schools. These include:

(a) Training teachers to incorporate instructions about values in the classroom. The classroom can provide an environment whereby students can learn respect for each other's opinion, cooperative behavior and responsibility and concern for classmates. The www.responsiveclassroom.org website provides further information on how value instruction can be incorporated in the classroom.
(b) Encourage a caring community throughout the school. Teachers, staff, adminis-trators, and others can model respectful and caring behavior. See www.devstu. org for information on how to create a sense of community within schools;
(c) Enforce positive discipline. Yael and Leishmen note that schools can pro-mote prosocial behavior by using positive discipline such as making clear expectations and modeling prosocial behavior.

Evidence-Based Practices for Increasing Prosocial Behavior

One evidence-based program for increasing prosocial behavior is Second Step (Frey, Nolan, Van Schoiack-Edstrom, & Hirschstein, 2005). This program increases prosocial behavior while at the same time reducing aggressive behavior and is listed on SAMHSA National Register of Evidenced Based Program and Practices. The program designed for children from 4 to 14 years of age uses social learning theory, empathy theory, and social information processing theories as the foundation for increasing prosocial behavior. The program comprises an in-school component, parental training, and skill development. Participants learn how to manage their emotions and how to make good decisions. There are two curriculums – one for preschool through fifth grade (with 20–25 sessions) and one for sixth through ninth graders (15 lessons in year one and eight sessions in the following 2 years). See http://www.cfchildren.org for further information or contact Claudia Glaze at Committee for Children, 568 First Avenue South, Suite 600, Seattle, WA 98104–2804, Phone: (206) 438–6500.

Preventing Teen Partner and Dating Violence

The Center for Disease Control, National Center for Injury Prevention and Control recognizes the importance of respect in preventing dating and partner violence. It created an interactive web program for adolescents (11–14 years of age), their parents, and others called *Choose Respect*. *Choose Respects* helps adolescents form healthy relationships before violence starts. The program involves (1) providing effective messages for adolescents, parents, teachers, and others that encourage adolescents to treat themselves and others with respect; (2) providing information for readers to learn about positive relationships; (3) increasing adolescent's ability to recognize abusive relationships; and (4) providing resources for preventing dating violence. The program has different types of material that can be accessed via the internet, including eCards, posters, online games, quizzes, etc. There are also television and radio spots, and press kits on how to use the media to highlight the message.

Resources

"Choose Respect" is a 30-minute video of stories from teens who have been in abusive relationships along with parents and professionals who have seen these relationships. The video was developed by the Centers for Disease Control. People in the video describe their experiences with physical and emotional abuse so that these can be spotted by others in relationships. There is also a 13-minute video that is targeted just for teens. http://www.chooserespect.org/scripts/materials/videos/videos.asp.

The Safe space web site has several resources devoted to stopping teen partner and domestic violence. The site includes information on legal rights, safety planning, and how to help a friend. http://www.thesafespace.org/index.htm.

School-based violence prevention programs: *A Resource Manual for Preventing Violence against Girls and Young Women* is a web site that identifies several school-based resources for preventing violence against girls and young women. This site may be helpful to school administrators, teachers, researchers, community organizations, and others interested in preventing violence among girls. The site provides a review of programs that target violence against women along with resources. The site address is: http://www.ucalgary.ca/resolve/violenceprevention/English/index.htm.

Elias, M., Zins, J. E. (2004). *Bullying, Peer Harassment, and Victimization in the Schools: The Next Generation of Prevention.* New York: Haworth. This book identifies risk and protective factors and provides practitioners with specific, evidence-based guidelines for preventing violence.

Concluding Comments

This book has described the realities and the experiences of African American adolescent girls with an emphasis on ways in which we can support her psychological, social, and physical development. The intent was to highlight her resiliencies and her strengths. Self-attributes such as high confidence, self-complexity, high achievement orientation, and androgynous gender roles are strengths and a foundation for positive growth and development. Her family is important to her well-being and further supports her growth and development through positive parental communication and monitoring. Peers and friends provide opportunities in which her relational and intimacy needs can be met. Communities further support her positive growth and development through after-school programming and educational and recreational activities. The "Recommendation and Resource" section of each chapter provides suggestions that should be useful for almost anyone working with and/or interested in African American girls' development.

At the same time, the intent was not to gloss over the problems and the realities of her world. At least one-third live in poverty, there remain high rates of pregnancy and sexually transmitted infections, many engage in poor health and fitness behaviors, and the neighborhood in which she lives is often underresourced. These situations have also been described in this book. My hope is that the reader has become more aware of her strengths and ways to prevent and reduce some of these problems.

In conclusion, African American girls are both unique and similar to other girls and to African American boys. Her attitudes and behaviors both converge and diverge with other groups. And just as she is affected by the context in which she lives to include friends, family, community, and school, she also exerts influence on these individuals and systems. Finally, while summary and generalized information have been presented, we must always be mindful of the heterogeneity and the individuality among African American girls.

References

Adelabu, D. H. (2008). Future time perspective, hope, and ethnic identity among African American adolescents. *Urban Education, 43*(3), 347–360.

Adelabu, D. H. (2007). Time perspective and school membership as correlates to academic achievement among African American adolescents. *Adolescence, 42*(167), 525–538.

Affenito, S., Thompson, D., Franko, R., Striegel-Moore, R., Daniels, S. R., Barton, B. A., et al. (2007). Longitudinal assessment of micronutrient intake among African-American and White girls: The national heart, lung, and blood institute growth and health study. *Journal of the American Dietetic Association, 107*(7), 1113–1123.

Akinbami, L. (2006). *Asthma prevalence, health care use and mortality: United States, 2003–2005.* Office of Analysis and Epidemiology, National Center for Health Statistics.

Akinbami, L. J. & Schoendorf, K. C. (2002). Trends in childhood asthma: Prevalence, health care utilization, and mortality. *Pediatrics, 110*, 315–322.

Alexander, K. L. (1997). Public schools and the public good. *Social Forces, 76(1)*, 1–30.

Allison, K. W., Burton, L., Marshall, S., Perez-Febles, A., Yarrington, J., Kirsh, L. B., et al. (1999). Life experiences among urban adolescents: examining the role of context. *Child Development, 70*(4), 1017–1029.

Alvy, K. (1994). *Parent training today: A social necessity.* Studio City, CA: Center for the Improvement of Child Caring, 1–377.

Amato, P. (1994). Father-child relations, mother-child relations, and offspring well-being in early adulthood. *Journal of Marriage and the Family, 56*, 1031–1042.

Anderson, S. E. & Must, A. (2005). Interpreting the continued decline in the average age of menarche: Results from two nationally representative surveys of US girls studied 10 years apart. *Journal of Pediatrics, 147*, 753–760.

Annunziata, D., Hogue, A., Faw, L., & Liddle, H. A. (2006). Family functioning and school success in at-risk, inner-city adolescents. *Journal of Youth and Adolescence, 35*(1), 105–113.

Archer, J. (2001). A strategic approach to aggression. *Social Development, 10*, 267–271.

Ashcraft, A. (2004). *Qualitative Investigation of Urban African American Mother/Daughter Communication about Relationships and Sex.* Unpublished doctoral dissertation, Virginia Commonwealth University.

Ashcraft, A. M. & Belgrave, F. Z. (2004). Gender identity development in urban African American girls. In J. W. Lee (Eds.), *Gender roles.* Hauppauge, NY: Nova Science Publishers.

Asthma Allergy Foundation of American (2008). Retrieved October 10, 2008 from http://www.aafa.org/index.cfm

Baldry, A. C. & Farrington, D. P. (2000). Bullies and delinquents: Personal characteristics and parental styles. *Journal of Community & Applied Social Psychology, 10*(1), 17–31.

Ball, J., Armistead, L., & Austin, B. (2003). The relationship between religiosity and adjustment among African American, female, urban adolescents. *Journal of Adolescene, 26(4)*, 431–446.

Baly, I. (1989). Career and vocational development of Black youth. In R. L. Jones (Ed.) *Black Adolescents*, (pp. 249–265). Berkeley, CA: Cobb & Henry Publishers.

Baranowski, T., Baranowski, J., Cullen, K., Thompson, D., Nicklas, T., & Zakeri, I. F. (2003). The fun, food, and fitness project (FFFP): The Baylor GEMS pilot study. *Ethnicity and Disease*, 13(Suppl. 1), S30–S39.

Baumeister, R. F. (1999). *The self in social psychology*. Philadelphia: Taylor & Frances.

Begley, E., Crosby R. A., DiClemente, R. J., et al. (2003). Older partners and STD prevalence among pregnant African American teens. *Sexually Transmitted Diseases*, 30(3), 211–213.

Belgrave, F. Z. & Allison, K. (2006). *African American Psychology*, 2nd ed. Thousand Oaks: CA: Sage Publications, Inc.

Belgrave, F. Z. & Allison, K. W. (2008). *African American Psychology: From Africa to America*, 2nd ed. Thousand Oaks: CA: Sage Publications, Inc.

Belgrave, F. Z., Brome, D., & Hampton, C. (2000). The contributions of Africentric values and racial identity to the prediction of drug knowledge, attitudes and use among African American youth. *Journal of Black Psychology*, 26(4), 386–401.

Belgrave, F. Z., Chase-Vaughn, G., Gray, F., Dixon-Addison, J., & Cherry, V. R. (2000). The effectiveness of a culture and gender specific intervention for increasing resiliency among African American pre-adolescent females. *Journal of Black Psychology*, 26(2), 123–147.

Belgrave, F. Z., Cherry, V., Butler, D., & Townsend, T. (2008). *Sister of Nia: A Cultural Enrichment Program to Empower African American Girls*. Chicago, IL: Research Press.

Belgrave, F. Z., Corneille, M. A., Nasim, A., Fitzgerald, A., & Lucas, V. (2008). An evalution of an Enhanced Sisters Informing Sisters about Topics on AIDS (SISTA) HIV Prevention Curriculum: The Role of Drug Education. *Journal of HIV/AIDS & Social Services*, 7(4), 313–327.

Belgrave, F. Z., Reed, M. C., & Plybon, L. E. (2004). The impact of a culturally enhanced drug prevention program on drug and alcohol refusal efficacy among urban African American girls. *Journal of Drug and Education*, 34(3), 267–279.

Belgrave, F. Z., Reed, M. C., & Plybon, L. E., Butler, D. S., Allison, K. W., & Davis, T. (2004). An evaluation of Sisters of Nia: A cultural program for African American girls. *The journal of Black Psychology*, 30(3), 329–343.

Bem, S. L. (1993). *The lenses of gender: Transforming the debate on sexual inequality*. New Haven: Yale.

Bilbarz, T. & Raftery, A. (1999). Family structure, educational attainment, and socioeconomic success: Rethinking the "pathology of matriarchy." *The American Journal of Sociology*, 105, 321–365.

Borawaski, E., Ievers-Landis, C., Lovegreen, L., & Trapl, E. (2003). Parental monitoring negotiated unsupervised time and parental trust: The role of perceived parenting practices in adolescent health risk behavior. *Journal of Adolescent Health*, 33(2), 60–70.

Boyd, K. (2003). *The effects of family influence and peer support on perceived self-efficacy for safe sex practices and drug refusal among African American adolescent girls in urban communities*. Unpublished doctoral dissertation, Virginia Commonwealth University, VA.

Boykin, A. W. & Toms, F. D. (1985). Black child socialization: A conceptual framework. In H. McAdoo & J. McAdoo (Eds.), *Black children* (pp. 33–51). Beverly Hills, CA: Sage.

Bradley, C. R. (1998). Child rearing in African American families: A study of the disciplinary practices of African American parents. *Journal of Multicultural Counseling and Development*, 26(4), 273–281.

Brausch, A. M. & Muehlenkamp, J. J. (2007). Body image and suicidal ideation in adolescents. *Body Image*, 4(2), 207–212.

Broderick, P. C. & Korteland, C. (2002). Coping style and depression in early adolescence: Relationships to gender, gender role, and implicit beliefs. *Sex Roles*, 46(7), 201–213.

Brown, C. (1997). Sex differences in the career development of urban African American adolescents. *Journal of Career Development*, 23, 295–304.

Buckley, T. R. & Carter, R. T. (2005). Black adolescent girls: Do gender role and racial identity impact their self-esteem? *Sex Roles*, 53(9–10), 647–661.

Burlew, K., Neely, D., & Johnson, C. (2000). Drug attitudes, racial identity, and alcohol use among African American adolescents. *Journal of Black Psychology*, 26, 402–420.

Burton, L. M. (2001). One step forward and two steps back: Neighborhoods, adolescent development, and unmeasured variables. In A. Booth & A. C. Crouter (Eds.), *Does it take a village? Community effects on children, adolescents, and families*. Mahwah, NJ: Lawrence Erlbaum Associates.

Bynum, M. S., Burton, E. T., & Best, C. (2007). Racism experiences and psychological functioning in African American college freshmen: Is racial socialization a buffer? *Cultural Diversity and Ethnic Minority Psychology, 13(1)*, 64–71.

Cash, T. F. & Pruzinsky, T. (1990). *Body images: Development, deviance, and change*. New York: Guilford Press.

Ceballo, R., McLoyd, V. C., & Toyokawa, T. (2004). The influence of neighborhood quality on adolescents' educational values and school effort. *Journal of Adolescent Research, 19*, 716–739.

Cecil, H. & Matson, S. C. (2006). Sexual victimization among African American adolescent females: Examination of the reliability and validity of the Sexual Experiences Survey. *Journal of Interpersonal Violence, 21(1)*, 89–104.

Centers for Disease Control. National Health & Nutrition Examination Survey (2006). Retrieved October 10, 2008 from http://www.cdc.gov/nchs/nhanes/nhanes20052006/nhanes05_06.htm.

Centers for Disease Control (1998). Youth Risk Behavior Surveillance: United States, 1997. *Morbidity & Mortality Weekly Report, 47*(SS3), 1–89.

Centers for Disease Control (2007). Cases of HIV infection and AIDS in the United States and Dependent Areas, 2005. *HIV/AIDS Surveillance Report, 17*, 1–46.

Centers for Disease Control (2008). Youth Risk Behavior Surveillance: United States, 2007. *Morbidity & Mortality Weekly Report, 57*(SS4), 1–131.

Centers for Disease Control and Prevention, National Center for Chronic Disease Prevention and Health Promotion. *Adolescent Reproductive Health*. Retrieved June 30, 2008, from http://www.cdc.gov/reproductivehealth/AdolescentReproHealth/index.htm.

Chaskin, R. J. (1998). *Defining neighborhoods*. Retrieved September 2, 2008, from http://www.planning.org/casey/pdf/chaskin.pdf.

Cherry, V. R. & Belgrave, F. Z. (1999). *Project Naja, Final Report*. Rockville, MD: Center for Substance Abuse Prevention.

Chiteji, N. & Hamilton, D. (2005). Family matters: Kin networks and asset accumulation. In M. Sherraden (Ed). *Inclusion in the American Dream: Assets, Poverty, and Public Policy*, (pp. 87). Oxford University Press.

Clark, T. T., Belgrave, F. Z. & Nasim, A. (2008). Risk and protective factors for substance use among urban African American adolescents considered high-risk. *Journal of Ethnicity in Substance Abuse, 7(3)*, 292–303.

Clark, T. T., Nguyen, A. B., & Belgrave, F. Z. (submitted). Risk and protective factors for alcohol and marijuana use among African American rural and urban adolescents. *Journal of Child and Adolescent Substance Abuse*.

Coard, S. I. & Sellers, R. M. (2005). African American families as a context for racial socialization. In V. Mcloyd, N. Hill, & K. Dodge (Eds.) *African American Family Life: Ecological and Cultural Diversity* (Chapter 13). Guilford Press, Inc.

Cohen, C. J. & Dawson, M. C. (1993). Neighborhood poverty and African American politics. *American Political Science Review, 87(2)*, 286–302.

Cohen, D., Farley, T., Taylor, S., Martin, D., & Schuster, M. (2002). When and where do youths have sex? The potential role of adult supervision. *Pediatrics, 110(6)*, 1239.

Coleman, M., Ganon, L. H., Clark, J. M., & Madsen, R. (1989). Parenting perceptions in rural and urban families: Is there a difference? *Journal of Marriage and Family, 51*, 329–335.

Coley, R. L. (2003). Daughter-father relationships and adolescent psychosocial functioning in low income African American families. *Journal of Marriage and the Family, 65*, 867–875.

Collins, R., Elliott, M., Berry, S., Kanouse, D., Kunkely, D., Hunter, S., & Miu, A. (2004). Watching sex on television predicts adolescent initiation of sexual behavior. *Pediatrics, 114(3)*, 45–57.

Congressional Food Stamp Challenge (2007). *U.S members of Congress live on a food stamp budget*. Retrieved July 31, 2008, from http://foodstampchallenge.typepad.com/.

Connolly, J. & Johnson, A. M. (1996). Adolescents' romantic relationships and the structure and quality of their interpersonal ties. *Personal Relationships, 3*, 185–195.

Constantine, M. G., Alleyne, V. L., Wallace, B. C., & Franklin-Jackson, D. C. (2006). Africentric cultural values: Their relation to positive mental health in African American adolescent girls. *Journal of Black Psychology, 32*(2), 141–154.

Cook, D. A. & Wiley, C. Y. (2000). Psychotherapy with members of African American Churches and spiritual traditions. In R. P. Scott & A. E. Bergin (Eds.). Handbook of Psychotherapy and Religious Diversity (pp. 39–396). Washington, DC: American Psychological Association.

Cooper, S. M. & Guthrie, B. (2007). Ecological influences on health-promoting and health-compromising behaviors. *Family Community Health, 30*(1), 29–41.

Corneille, M. A., Ashcraft, A. M., & Belgrave, F. Z. (2005). What's culture got to do with it? Prevention programs for African American adolescent girls. *Journal of Health Care for the Poor and Underserved, 16(2, SupplB)*, 38–47.

Corneille, M. A. & Belgrave, F. Z. (2007). Ethnic identity, neighborhood risk, and adolescent drug and sex attitudes and refusal efficacy: The urban African American girls' experience. *Journal of Drug Education, 37*, 177–190.

Costigan, C. L., Cauce, A. M., & Etchison, K. (2007). Changes in African American mother-daughter relationships during adolescence: Conflict, autonomy, and warmth. In B. J. R. Leadbeater & N. Way (Eds.), *Urban girls revisited: Building strengths* (pp. 177–201). New York, NY: New York University Press.

Cottrell, L. (2003). Parent and adolescent perceptions of parental monitoring and adolescent risk involvement. *Science & Practice, 3*(3), 279–295.

Crick, N. R., Bigbee, M. A., & Howes, C. (1996). Gender differences in children's normative beliefs about aggression: How do I hurt thee? Let me count the ways. *Child Development, 67*, 1003–1014.

Crick, N. R. & Grotpeter, J. K. (1995). Relational aggression, gender, and social-psychological adjustment. *Child Development, 66*(3), 710–722.

Crosby, R. A., DiClemente, R. J., Wingood, G. M., Harrington, K., Davies, S., & Oh, M. K. (2002). Activity of African-American female teenagers in black organizations is associated with STD/HIV protective behaviors: A prospective analysis. *Journal of Epidemiology & Community Health, 56*(7), 549–550.

Crosby, R. A., DiClemente, R. J., Wingood, G. A., Lang, D. L., & Harrington, K. (2003). Infrequent parental monitoring predicts sexually transmitted infections among low income African American female adolescents. *Archives of Pediatrics and Adolescent Medicine, 157*, 169–173.

Cunningham, M. & Thornton, A. (2007). Direct and indirect influences of parents' marital instability on children's attitudes toward cohabitation in young adulthood. *Journal of Divorce and Remarraige, 46(3)*, 125–143.

D'Augelli, A. R. (2006). Developmental and contextual factors and mental health among lesbian, gay, and bisexual youths. In A. M. Omoto & S. Howard (eds.). *Sexual orientation and mental health: Examining identity and development in lesbian, gay, and bisexual people* (pp. 37–53). Washington, DC: American Psychological Association.

Daves, J. A. (1995). Addressing television sexuality with adolescents. *Pediatric Annals, 24*, 79–82.

Davies, S. L., DiClemente, R. J., Wingood, G. M. (2003). Pregnancy desire among disadvantaged African American adolescent females. *American Journal of Health Behavior, 27*(1), 55–62.

Davies, P. T. & Windle, M. (2000). Middle adolescents' dating pathways and psychological adjustment. *Merrill-Palmer Quarterley, 46(1)*, 90–118.

Deater-Deckard, K., Dodge, K. A., Bates, J. E., & Pettit, G. S. (2004). Ethnic differences in the link between physical discipline and adolescent externalizing behaviors. *Journal of Child Psychology and Psychiatry, 45(4)*, 801–812.

Diamond, M. (2002). Sex and gender are different: Sexual identity and gender identity are different. *Clinical Child Psychology and Psychiatry, 7*(3), 320–334.

DiClemente, R. & Wingood, G. (2001). Parental monitoring: Association with adolescents' risk behavior. *Pediatrics, 107*(6), 1363–1368.

Dittus, P. J. & Jaccard, J. (2000). Adolescents' perceptions of maternal disapproval of sex: Relationship to sexual outcomes. *Journal of Adolescent Health, 26*, 268–278.

Dittus, P., Jaccard, J., & Gordon, V. V. (1997). The impact of African American fathers on adolescent sexual behavior. *Journal of Youth and Adolescence, 26*(4), 445–465.

Dixon, R., Gill, J., & Adair, V. (2003). Exploring paternal influences on the dieting behavior of adolescent girls. *The Journal of Treatment & Prevention, 11*(1), 39–50.

Dolcini, M. M. & Adler, N. E. (2004). Perceived competence, peer group affiliation, and risk behavior among early adolescents. *Health Psychology, 13*(6), 496–506.

Dorius, G. L, Heaton, T. B., & Steffen, P. (1993). Adolescent life events and their association with the onset of sexual intercourse. *Youth & Society, 25*(1), 3–23.

Dornelas, E., Pattern, C., Fischer, E., Decker, P., Offord, K., Barbagallo, J., et al. (2005). Ethnic variation in socioenvironmental factors that influence adolescent smoking. *Journal of Adolescent Health, 36*(3), 170–177.

Duncan, S. C., Duncan, T. E., & Strycker, L. A. (2002). A multilevel analysis of neighborhood context and youth alcohol and drug problems. *Prevention Science, 3*(2), 125–133.

Eagly, A. H. & Steffen, V. J. (2000). Gender stereotypes stem from the distribution of women and men into social roles. In C. Stanger (Ed.) *Stereotypes and prejudice*. Philadelphia, PA: Taylor & Frances.

East, P. L. (1998). Racial and ethnic differences in girls' sexual, marital and birth expectations. *Journal of Marriage and the Family, 60*(1), 150–162.

Ellis, B. J., Bates, J. E., Dodge, K. A., Fergusson, M. M., Horwood, J., Petit, G. S., & Woodward, L. (2003). Does father absence place daughters at special risk for early sexual activity and teenage pregnancy. *Child Development, 74*(3), 801–821.

Espelage, D. L., Bosworth, K., & Simon, T. R. (2000). Examining the social context of bullying behaviors in early adolescence. *Journal of Counseling and Development, 78*, 326–333.

Esposito, L. E. (2008). The role of empathy, anger management and normative beliefs about aggression in bullying among urban, African-American middle school children (Doctoral dissertation, Virginia Commonwealth University, 2008). *Dissertation Abstracts International, 68*(11-B), 7708.

Federal Interagency Forum on Child and Family Statistics (2007). *America's children: Key national indicators of well-being 2007*. Washington, D.C., U.S. Government Printing Office.

Feshbach, N. D. (1997). Empathy: The formative years. Implications for clinical practice. In A. C. Bohart & L. S. Greenberg (Eds.), *Empathy reconsidered: Directions for psychotherapy* (pp. 33–59). Washington, DC: American Psychological Association.

Festinger, L. (1954). A theory of social comparison processes. *Human Relations, 7*, 117–140.

Freedner, N., Freed, L. H., Yang, Y. W., Austin, S. B. (2002). Dating violence among gay, lesbian, and bisexual adolescents: Results from a community survey. *Journal of Adolescent Health, 31*, 469–474.

Frey, K. S., Nolen, S. B., Van Schoiack-Edstrom, L., & Hirschstein, M. K. (2005). Effect of a school-based social-emotional competence program: Linking children's goals, attributions, and behavior. *Applied Developmental Psychology, 26*, 171–200.

Foley, L. A., Evancic, C., & Karnik, K. (1995). Date rape: Effects of race assailant and victim and gender of subjects on perceptions. *Journal of Black Psychology, 21*(1), 6–18.

Fordham, S. & Ogbu, J. (1986). Black students and school success: Coping with the burden of "acting white." *Urban Review, 18*(3), 176–206.

Foster, J. D., Kupermine, G. P., & Price, A. W. (2004). Gender differences in posttraumatic stress and related symptoms among inner-city minority youth exposed to community violence. *Journal of Youth and Adolescence, 33*(1), 59–69.

Franko, D. L., Striegel-Moore, R. H., Bean, J., Tamer, R., Kraemer, H. C., Dohm, F. A., et al. (2005). Psychosocial and health consequences of adolescent depression in black and white young adult women. *Health Psychology, 24*, 586–593.

Fuligni, A., Eccles, J., Barber, B., & Clements, P. (2001). Early adolescent peer orientation and adjustment during high school. *Developmental Psychology, 37*, 28–36.

Gaines, S. O. & Brennan, K. A. (2001). Establishing and maintaining satisfaction in multicultural relationships. In J. Harvey & A. Wenzel (Eds.) *Close Romantic Relationships: Maintenance and Enhancement* (pp. 237–252). Lawrence Erlbaum Associates.

Garcia-Coll, C., Meyer, E., & Brillon, L. (1995). Ethnic and minority parenting. In M. Bornstein (Ed.), *Handbook of parenting: Biology and Ecology of Parenting* (pp. 189–209). Hillsdale, NJ: Lawrence Erlbaum Associates.

Garrison, C. Z., Schoenbach, V. J., Schluchter, M. D., & Kaplan, B. H. (1987). Life events in early adolescence. *Journal of the American Academy of Child and Adolescent Psychiatry, 26*, 865–872.

Ge, X., Kim, I. J., Brody, G. H., Conger, R. D., Simons, R. L., Gibbons, F. X. et al. (2003). It's about timing and change: pubertal transition effects on symptoms of major depression among African American youths. *Developmental Psychology, 39(3)*, 430–439.

Goldston, D. B., Molock, S. D., & Whitbeck, L. B. (2008). Cultural considerations in adolescent suicide prevention and psychosocial treatment. *American Psychologist, 63*(1), 14–31.

Goodkind, S., Ng, I., & Sarri, R. C. (2006). The impact of sexual abuse in the lives of young women involved or at risk for involvement with the juvenile justice system. *Violence Against Women, 12(5)*, 456–477.

Goodwin, R. (1990). Sex differences among partner preferences: Are the sexes really very similar? *Sex Roles, 23*, 501–513.

Gordon, M. K. (2004). Media images of women and African American girl's sense of self. *Dissertation Abstracts International, 65*(6-B), 3197.

Gordon-Larsen, P., Griffiths, P., Bentley, M. E., Ward, D. S., Kelsey, K., Shields, K. et al. (2004). Barriers to physical activity: Qualitative data on caregiver-daughter perceptions and practices. *American Journal of Preventive Medicine, 27*(3), 218–223.

Graber, J. A. & Sontag, L. M. (2006). Puberty and girls' sexuality: Why hormones are not the complete answer. *New Directions for Child & Adolescent Development, 112*, 23–38.

Graham, Lansford, J. E., Graham, S., Taylor, A. Z., & Hudley, C. (1998). Exploring achievement values among ethnic minority early adolescents. *Journal of Educational Psychology, 90*(4), 606–620.

Granberg, E. M., Simons, R. L., & Gibbons, F. X. (2008). The relationship between body size and depressed mood: Findings from a sample of African American middle school girls. *Youth and Society, 39*(3), 294–315.

Greene, M. L. & Way, N. (2005). Self-esteem trajectories among ethnic minority adolescents: A growth curve analysis of the patterns and predictors of change. *Journal of Research on Adolescence, 15*(2), 151–178.

Gruenewalkd, P. J., Millar, A., Ponicki, W. R., & Brinkley, G. (2000). Physical and economic access to alcohol. In R. A. Wilson & M. C. Dufour (Eds.), *The epidemiology of alcohol problems in small geographic areas* (NIH Pub. No. 00-4357; pp. 163–212). Bethesda, MD: NIH.

Grunbaum, J. A., Kann, L., Kinchen, S. A., Williams, B., Ross, J. G., Lowry, R., et al. (2002). Youth Risk Behavior Surveillance: United States 2001. *Morbidity and Mortality Weekly Report, 51*(SS04), 1–64.

Guthrie, B. J., Young, A. M., Williams, D. R., Boyd, C. J., & Kintner, E. K. (2002). African American girls' smoking habits and day-to-day experiences with racial discrimination. *Nursing Research, 51*(3), 183–190.

Halpern, C. T., Young, M. L., Waller, M. W., Martin, G. L., & Cooper, L. L. (2004). Prevalence of partner violence in same-sex romantic and sexual relationships in a national sample of adolescents. *Journal of Adolescent Health, 35*, 124–131.

Hamilton, B., Martin, J. A., & Ventura, S. J. (2007). Births: Preliminary Date for 2006. Division of Vital Statistics, National Vital Statistical Report, *56*(7), Dec 5, 2007.

Hamm, J. V. (2000). Do birds of a feather flock together? The variable bases for African American, Asian American, and European American adolescents' selection of similar friends. *Developmental Psychology, 36*(2), 209–219.

Haney, T. J. (2007). "Broken windows" and self-esteem: Subjective understandings of neighborhood poverty and disorder. *Social Science Research, 36*, 968–994.

Hansen, S. L. (1977). Dating choices of high school students. *Family Coordinator, 26*(2), 133–138.

Harper, G. W., Gannon, C., Watson, S. E., Catania, J. A., & Dolcini, M. M. (2004). The role of close friends in African American adolescents' dating and sexual behavior. *The Journal of Sex Research, 41*(4), 351–362.

Harris, A. C. (1996). African American and Anglo-American gender identities: An empirical study. *Journal of Black Psychology, 22*(2), 182–194.

Harris-Peterson, S. (2006). The importance of fathers contextualizing sexual risk taking in low-risk African American girls. *The Journal of Human Behavior in the Social Environment, 13*(3), 67–83.

Hart, D. & Fegley, S. (1995). Prosocial behavior and caring in adolescence: Relations to self-understanding and social judgment. *Child Development, 66*(5), 1346–1359.

Hartup, W. W. & Stevens, N. (1999). Friendship and adaptation across the life span. *Current Directions in Psychological Science, 8(3)*, 76–79.

Hechman, J. J. & LaFontaine, P. A. (2007). The American high school graduation rate: Trends levels. Institute for the Study of Labor. Accessed January 5, 2009, at http://ftp.iza.org/dp3216.pdf.

Hedgepeth, V. (2008). *Effects of the quality of parent-child relationships on body image satisfaction and image acculturation among African American girls: The mediating role of racial identity.* Unpublished Dissertation, Virginia Commonwealth University, 2008.

Hellenga, K., Aber, M. S., & Rhodes, J. E. (2002). African American adolescent mother's vocational aspiration-expectation gap: Individual, social, and environmental influences. *Psychology of Women, 26*, 200–212.

Helms, J. (1990). *Black and White Racial Identity: Theory, Research, and Practice.* New York: Greenwood Press.

Hill, M. E. (2002). Skin color and the perception of attractiveness among African Americans: Does gender make a difference? *Social Psychology Quarterly, 65*(1), 77–91.

Hill, R. B. (1998). Understanding black family functioning: A holistic perspective. *Journal of Comparative Family Studies, 29*(1), 15–25.

Hobbs, R. (1997). Literacy for the information age. In J. Flood, S. B. Heath, & D. Lapp (Eds.), *Handbook of research on teaching literacy through the communicative and visual arts* (pp. 7–14). New York: Simon Schuster Macmillan.

Hollist, D. R. & McBroom, W. H. (2006). Family structure, family tension, and self-reported marijuana use: A research finding of risky behavior among youths. *Journal of Drug Issues, 36*(4), 975–998.

Honora, D. T. (2002). The relationship of gender and achievement to future outlook among African American adolescents. *Adolescence, 37*(146), 300–316.

Howard, D. E., Wang, M. Q., & Yan, F. (2007). Prevalence and psychosocial correlates of forced sexual intercourse among U.S. high school adolescents. *Adolescence, 42*(168), 629–643.

Howard, D. E., Wang, M. Q., & Yan, F. (2007). Psychological factors associated with reports of physical dating violence among U.S. adolescent females. *Adolescence, 42*(166), 311–324.

Howard, D. W., Kaljee, L., Rachuba, L. T., & Cross, S. I. (2003). Coping with youth violence: Assessments by minority parents in public housing. *American Journal of Health Behavior, 27*(5), 483–492.

Hrabowski, F. A., Maton, K. I., Greene, M. L. & Greif, G. L. (2002). *Overcoming the odds: Raising academically successful African American young women.* New York, NY: Oxford University Press.

Hudley, C. & Graham, S. (2001). Stereotypes of achievement striving among early adolescents. *Social Psychology of Education, 5*(2), 201–224.

Hughes, D. (2003). Correlates of African Americana and Latino parents' messages to children about ethnicity and race: A comparative study of racial socialization. *American Journal of Community Psychology, 31(1–2)*, 15–33.

Hunger, M. L. (2002). 'If you're light you're alright': Light skin as social capital for women of color. *Gender & Society, 16*(2), 175–193.

Hurley, E. A., Boykin, A. W., & Allen, B. A. (2005). Communal versus individual learning of a math-estimation task: African American children the culture of learning contexts. *Journal of Psychology: Interdisciplinary and Applied, 139*(6), 513–527.

Jaccard, J., Dittus, P. J., & Gordon, V. V. (1998). Parent-adolescent congruency in reports of adolescent sexual behavior and in communications about sexual behavior. *Child Development, 69*(1), 247–261.

Jagers, R. J. & Smith, P. (1996). Further explanation of the spirituality scale. *Journal of Black Psychology, 22*, 429–442.

Jemmott, J. B., Jemmott, L. S., & Fong, G. T. (1992). Reductions in HIV risk-associated sexual behaviors among Black male adolescents: Effects of an AIDS prevention intervention. *American Journal of Public Health, 82*, 372–377.

Joint Center for Political and Economic Studies. (2001, October). *Marriage and African Americans*. Retrieved August 28, 2008, from http://www.jointcenter.org/DB/factsheet/marital.htm.

Jones, J. (2003). TRIOS: A psychological theory of the African legacy in American culture. *Journal of Social Issues, 59*(1), 217–243.

Jones, D. C. & Crawford, J. K. (2005). The peer appearance culture during adolescence: Gender and body mass variations. *Journal of Youth and Adolescence, 35(2)*, 629–636.

Jones, L. R., Frieds, E., & Danish, S. J. (2007). Gender and ethnic differences in body image and opposite sex figure preferences of rural adolescents. *Body Image, 4(1)*, 103–108.

Kaestle, C. E., Halpern, C. T., & Brown, J. D. (2007). Music videos, pro wrestling, and acceptance of date rape among middle school males and females: An exploratory analysis. *Journal of Adolescent Health, 40*(2), 185–187.

Kaiser Family Foundation (2001). Teens and sex: The Role of Popular TV [*Fact Sheet*]. Menlo Park, CA: The Foundation.

Kegler, M. C., Oman, R. F., Vesely, S. K., McLeroy, K.. R., Aspy, C. B., Rodine, S. et al. (2005). Relationships among youth assets and neighborhood and community resources. *Health Education and Behavior, 32(3)*, 380–397.

Kegler, M. C., Rodine, S., Marshall, L., Oman, R., & McLeroy, K. (2003). An asset-based youth development model for preventing teen pregnancy: Illustrations from the HEART of OKC Project. *Health Education, 103*(3), 131–144.

Kellar-DeMers, J. (2001). The relationship of father-daughter attachment to personality attributes and self-esteem in adolescent girls. *Dissertation Abstracts International, 62*(3-B).

Kelly, A. M., Wall, M., & Eisenberg, M. E. (2005). Adolescent girls with high body satisfaction: Who are they and what can they teach us? *Journal of Adolescent Health, 37*(5), 391–396.

Kenny, J. W., Reinholtz, C., & Angelini, R. J. (1997). Ethnic differences in childhood and adolescent sexual abuse and teenage pregnancy. *Journal of Adolescent Health, 21(1)*, 3 10.

Kerpelman, J. L, Eryigit, S., & Stephens, C. J. (2008). African American adolescents' future education orientation: Associations with self-efficacy, ethnic identity, and perceived parental support. *Journal of Youth and Adolescence, 37(8)*, 997–1008.

Kerpelman, J. L., Shoffner, M. F., & Ross-Griffin, S. (2002). African American mothers' and daughters' beliefs about possible selves ad their strategies for reaching the adolescents' future academic and career goals. *Journal of Youth and Adolescence, 31(4)*, 289–302.

Kidron, Y., & Fleischman, S. (2006). Research matters/ Promoting adolescents' prosocial behavior. *Teaching the Tweens, 63(7)*, 90–91.

Kids Source (1998, August 19). *Teenage girls today more independent, yet lack self-esteem*. Retrieved July 17, 2008, from http://www.kidsource.com/kidsource/content4/teenage.girls.esteem.news.html

Kim, S. & Glynn, N. W. (2004, August). *What we know about obesity development during adolescence. Findings from the NHLBI growth and health study.* Presented at the Predictors of Obesity, Weight Gain, Diet, and Physical Activity Workshop, Bethesda, MD.

Kimm, S., Glynn, N. W., Kriska, A. M., Barton, B. A., Kronsberg, S. S., Daniels, S. R., et al. (2002). Decline in the physical activity in black girls and white girls during adolescence, *The New England Journal of Medicine, 347*, 709–715.

Klesges, R. C., Obarzanek, K., Klesges, L. M., Stockton, M. B., Beech, B. M., Murray, D. M., et al. (2008). Memphis girl's health enrichment multi-site studies (GEMS) phase 2: Design and baseline. *Contemporary Clinical Trials, 29*(1), 42–55.

Kliewer, W. (2006). Violence exposure and cortisol responses in urban youth. *International Journal of Behavioral Medicine, 13*(2), 109–120.

Kliewer, W., Wilson, D. K., & Plybon, L. E. (2002). Gender differences in the relation between neighborhood quality and cardiovascular reactivity in African American adolescents. *Journal of Applied Social Psychology, 32*(4), 865–884.

Kosterman, R., Haggerty, K., Spoth, R., & Redmond, C. (2004). Unique influence of mothers and fathers on their children's antisocial behavior. *Journal of Marriage and Family, 66*, 762–778.

Kulig, K., Brenner, N., & McManus, T. (2003). Sexual activity and substance use among adolescents by category of physical activity plus team sports participation. *Archives of Pediatrics & Adolescent Medicine, 157*(9), 905–912.

Laflin, M. T., Wang, J., & Barry, M. (2008). A longitudinal study of adolescent transition from virgin to nonvirgin status. *Journal of Adolescent Health, 42*(3), 228–236.

Lambert, S. F., Brown, T. L., Phillips, C. M., & Ialongo, N. S. (2004). The relationships between perceptions of neighborhood characteristics and substance use among urban African American adolescents. *American Journal of Community Psychology, 34*(3–4), 205–218.

Le, T. N., Tov, W., & Taylor, J. (2007). Religiousness and depressive symptoms in five ethnic adolescent groups. *International Journal for the Psychology of Religion, 17*(3), 209–232.

Lenhart, A., Madden, M., MacGill, A. R., & Smith, A. (2007). *Teens and social media.* Internet and America Life Project. Washington, DC. Retrieved January 6, 2009, from http://www.pewinternet.org/pdfs/PIP_Teens_Social_Media_Final.pdf.

Li, X., Stanton, B., & Pack, R. (2002). Risk and protective factors associated with gang involvement among urban African American adolescents. *Youth & Society, 34*(2), 172–194.

Linville, P. W. (1985). Self-complexity and affective extremity: Don't put all of your eggs in one cognitive basket. *Social Cognition, 3*, 94–120.

Littlefield, M. B. (2008). The media as a system of racilization: Exploring images of African American women and the new racism. *American Behavioral Scientist, 51*(5), 675–685.

Loeb, T. B., Williams, J. K., Carmona, J. V., Rivkin, I., Wyatt, G. E., et al. (2002). Child sexual abuse: Associations with the sexual functioning of adolescents and adults. *Annual Review of Sex Research, 13*, 307–345.

Longmore, M. A., Manning, W. D., & Giordano, P. C. (2001). Preadolescent parenting strategies and teens' dating and sexual initiation: A longitudinal analysis. *Journal of Marriage and Family, 63*, 322–335.

MacQueen, K.M., McLellan, E., Metzger, D.S., Kegeles, S., Strauss, R.P., Scotti, R. et al. (2001). What is community? An evidence-based definition for participatory public health. *American Journal of Public Health, 91*(12), 1929–1938.

Magnus, K. B. & Cowen, E. L. (1999). Parent-child relationship qualities and child adjustment in highly stressed urban Black and White families. *Journal of Community Psychology, 27*(1), 55–71.

Marcus, M. T., Walker, T., Swint, J. M., Smith, B. P., Brown, C., Busen, N., et al. (2004). Community-based participatory research to prevent substance abuse and HIV/AIDS in African American adolescents. *Journal of Interprofessional Care, 18*(4), 348–359.

Marsiglia, F., Kulis, S., & Hecht, M. L. (2001). Ethnic labels and ethnic identity as predictors of drug use among middle school students in the southwest. *Journal of Research on Adolescence, 11*, 21–48.

168   References

McBride, C., Paikoff, R. L., & Grayson, H. (2003). Individual and familial influences on the onset of sexual intercourse among urban African American adolescents. *Journal of Consulting and Clinical Psychology, 71*(1), 159–167.

McCormick, D. P., Holder, B., Wetsel, M. A., & Cawthon, T. W. (2001). Spirituality and HIV disease: An integrated perspective. *The Journal of the Association of Nurses in AIDS Care, 21*, 58–65.

McLoyd, V. C. & Jozefowicz, D. M. H. (1996). Sizing up the future: Predictors of African American adolescent females' expectancies about their economic fortunes and family life outcomes. In B. Leadbeater & N. Way (Eds.), *Creating identities, resisting stereotypes: Urban adolescent girls* (pp. 355–379). New York: University Press.

McMahon, S. D., Wernsman, J., & Parnes, A. L. (2006). Understanding prosocial behavior: The impact of empathy and gender among African American Adolescents. *Journal of Adolescent Health, 39*(1), 135–137.

McNulty-Eitle, & Eitle, D. (2002). Just don't do it: High school sports participation and young female adult sexual behavior. *Sociology of Sport Journal, 19*(4), 403–418.

Mello, Z. R. & Swanson, D. P. (2007). Gender differences in African American adolescents' personal, educational, and occupational expectations and perceptions of neighborhood quality. *Journal of Black Psychology, 33*(2), 150–168.

Mickelson, R. A. & Greene, A. D. (2006). Connecting pieces of the puzzle: Gender differences in Black middle school students' achievement. *Journal of Negro Education, 75(1)*, 34–48.

Milevsky, A. & Levitt, M. J. (2004). Intrinsic and extrinsic religiosity in preadolescence and adolescence: Effect on psychological adjustment. *Mental Health, Religion & Culture, 7*(4), 307–321.

Milhausen, R. R., Crosby, R., Yarber, W. L., DiClemente, R. J., Wingood, G. M., & Ding, K. (2003). Rural and nonrural African American high school students and STD/HIV sexual risk behaviors. *American Journal of Health Behavior, 27*(4), 373–379.

Miller, B. C. (2002). Family influence on adolescent sexual and contraceptive behavior. *The Journal of Sex Research, 39*, 22–26.

Miller, J. (1991). The "self-in-relation." A theory of women's development. In J. S. Jordan, A. G. Kaplan, J. B. Miller, I. P. Stiver, & J. L. Surrey (Eds.), *Women's growth in connections* (pp. 202–220). New York: Guilford.

Miller, R. S. (1997). Inattentive and contented: Relationship commitment and attention to alternatives. *Journal of Personality and Social Psychology, 73(4)*, 758–766.

Miller, K. S., Forehand, R., & Kotchick, B. A. (1999). Adolescent sexual behavior in two ethnic minority samples: The role of family variables. *Journal of Marriage and the Family, 61*(1), 85–98.

Miller, B. C. & Moore, K. A. (1990). Adolescent sexual behavior, pregnancy, and parenting: Research through the 1980s. *Journal of Marriage and the Family, 52*, 1025–1044.

Mok, T. A. (1999). Asian American dating: Important factors in partner choice. *Cultural Diversity and Ethnic Minority Psychology, 5(2)*, 103–117.

Molnar, B. E., Roberts, A. L., Browne, A., Gardener, H., & Buka, S. L. (2004). What girls need: recommendations for preventing violence among urban girls in the U.S. *Social Science and Medicine, 60*(10), 2191–2204.

Morris, E. W. (2007). "Ladies" or "Loudies"? Perceptions and experiences of Black girls in classrooms. *Youth and Society, 38*(4), 490–515.

Mounts, N. S. & Steinberg, L. (1995). An ecological analysis of peer influence on adolescent's grade point average and drug use. *Developmental Psychology, 31*, 915–922.

Nainggolan, L. & Murata, P. (2007, January 12). Overweight girls at risk for cardiovascular disease. *MedScape.*

Nasim, A., Belgrave, F. Z., Corona, R., & Townsend, T. G. (2008). Predictors of tobacco and alcohol refusal efficacy for urban and rural adolescents. *Journal of Child and Adolescent Substance Use, 18(2)*, 221–242.

National Academy on an Aging Society (1999). *Chronic conditions*: A challenge for the 21st century. Retrieved October 10, 2008 from http://www.agingsociety.org/agingsociety/pdf/chronic.pdf

National Center for Health Statistics (NCHS, 2004). Nine million U.S. children diagnosed with asthma, new report finds. *Fact Sheet*. Retrieved October 10, 2008 from http://www.cdc.gov/nchs/pressroom/04news/childasthma.htm

National Health Interview Survey (2004). *Summary Health Statistics for US Children*. Retrieved October 10, 2008 from http://www.cdc.gov/nchs/data/series/sr_10/sr10_227.pdf

National Institute of Allergy and Infectious Diseases, National Institutes of Health. (2001). Asthma: A concern for minority populations. Retrieved October 10, 2008, from http://www.aafa.org/display.cfm?id=8&sub=42#_ftn17

National Institute of Child and Human Development. (2007). What is puberty. Retrieved October 10, 2008, from http://www.nichd.nih.gov/health/topics/puberty.cfm

National Institute of Diabetes and Digestive and Kidney Diseases, National Diabetes Statistics. (2007). Bethesda, MD: U.S. Department of Health and Human Services, National Institutes of Health, 2008. Retrieved October 10, 2008, from http://www.diabetes.niddk.nih.gov/dm/pubs/statistics/

Neblett, E. W., Philip, C. L., Cogburn, C. D., & Sellers, R. M. (2006). African American adolescents' discrimination experiences and academic achievement racial socialization as a cultural compensatory and protective factor. *Journal of Black Psychology, 32*(2), 199–218.

Negriff, S., Fung, M. T., & Trickeet, P. K. (2008). Self-rated pubertal development, depressive symptoms and delinquency: Measurement issues and moderation by gender and maltreatment. *Journal of Youth and Adolescence, 37*(6), 736–746.

Neighborhood. (2008). In *Wikepedia, the free encyclopedia*. Retrieved September 9, 2008, from http://en.wikipedia.org/wiki/Neighborhood

Nurmi, J. E. (2004). Socialization and self development: Channeling, selection, adjustment, and reflection. In R. Lerner & L. Steinberg (Eds.), *Handbook of adolescent psychology* (pp. 85–124). New York: Wiley.

Obeidallah , D., Brennan, R. T., Brooks-Gunn, J., & Earls, F. (2004). Links between pubertal timing and neighborhood contexts: Implications for girls' violent behavior. *Journal of the American Academy of Child & Adolescent Psychiatry, 43*(12), 1460–1468.

Ogbu, J. U. (1991). Cultural mode, identity, and literacy. In J. W. Stigler, R. A. Schweder, & G. Herdt (Eds.), *Cultural psychology* (pp. 520–541). New York: Cambridge University Press.

Olweus, D. (1993). *Bullying at School*. Cambridge: Blackwell Publishers.

Osborne, L. N. & Rhodes, J. E. (2001). The role of life stress and social support in the adjustment of sexually victimized pregnant and parenting minority adolescents. *American Journal of Community Psychology, 29*(6), 833–849.

O'Sullivan, L. F., et al. (2001). Mother-daughter communication about sex among urban African American and Latino families. *Journal of Adolescent Research, 16*, 269–292.

Oyserman, D., Bybee, D., & Terry, K. (2003). Gendered racial identity and involvement with school. *Self and Identity, 2*(4), 307–324.

Oyserman, D., Harrison, K., & Bybee, D. (2001). Can racial identity be promotive of academic efficacy? *International Journal of Behavioral Development, 25*(4), 379–385.

Oyserman, D., Terry, K., & Bybee, D. (2002). A possible selves intervention to enhance school involvement. *Journal of Adolescence, 25*, 313–326.

Pagano, M. E. & Hirsch, B. J. (2007). Friendships and romantic relationship of Black and White adolescents. *Journal of Child and Family Studies, 16*(3), 347–357.

Parke, R. & Buriel, R. (1998). Socialization in the family: Ethnic and ecological perspectives. In W. Damon & N. Eisenberg (Eds.), *Handbook of child psychology: Social, emotional and personality development, 5th ed., Vol. 3* (pp. 463–552). Hoboken, NJ: John Wiley & Sons, Inc.

Perez-Febles, A.M. (1999). Potential life course trajectories among African-American adolescent girls in urban neighborhoods. *Dissertation Abstracts International, 59*(8-B), 4480.

Phinney, J. S. & Kohatsu, E. L. (1997). Ethnic and racial identity development and mental health. In J. Schulenberg, J. L. Maggs, K. Hurrelmann (Eds.), *Health risks and development transitions during adolescence* (pp. 420–443). New York, NY: Cambridge University Press.

Pilgrim, C. L. (2006). Afrocentric education and the prosocial behavior of African American children. ETD Collection for Fordham University. Paper AAI3210276.

Pittman, L. D. & Chese-Lendale (2001). African American adolescent girls in impoverished communities: Parenting style and adolescent outcomes. *Journal of Research on Adolescence, 11*(2), 199–224.

Plybon, L. E., Edwards, L., Butler, D., Belgrave, F. Z., & Allison, K. W. (2003). Examining the link between neighborhood cohesion and school outcomes: The role of support coping among African American adolescent girls. *Journal of Black Psychology, 29*(4), 393–407.

Ponterotto, J.G., Utsey, S.O., & Pendersen, P.B. (2006). *Preventing prejudice: A guide for counselors, educators, and parents* (2nd ed.). Thousand Oaks, Ca: Sage Publications.

Puberty. (2008). In *Merriam-Webster Online Dictionary*. Retrieved July 31, 2008, from http://www.merriam-webster.com/dictionary/puberty

Quatman, T., Sampson, K., Robinson, C. & Watson, C. M. (2001). Academic, motivational, and emotional correlates of adolescent dating. *Genetic, Social, & General Psychology Monographs, 127*(2), 211–234.

Raiford, J. L., Wingood, G. M., & DiClemente, R. J. (2007). Prevalence, incidence, and predictors of dating violence: A longitudinal study of African American female adolescents. *Journal of Women's Health, 16*(6), 822–832.

Regan, P.C., Durbasula, R., Howell, L. Ureno, O., & Rea, M. (2004). Gender, ethnicity, and the developmental timing of first sexual and romantic experiences. *Social Behavior and Personality, 32(7)*, 667–676.

Reid, R. J., Peterson, N., Lowe, J. B., & Hughey, J. (2005). Tobacco outlet density and smoking prevalence: Does racial concentration matter? *Drugs, Education, Prevention, & Policy, 12*(3), 233–238.

Resnick, M. D., et al. (1997). Protecting adolescents from harm: Findings from the National Longitudinal Study on Adolescent Health. *Journal of American Medical Association, 278*, 823–832.

Ricciuti, H. N. (2004). Single parenthood, achievement, and problem behavior in white, black and Hispanic children. *The Journal of Educational Research, 97(4)*, 96–206.

Richards, M., Gitelson, I., Petersen, A., & Hurtig, A. (1991). Adolescent personality in girls and boys: The role of mothers and fathers. *Psychology of Women Quarterly, 15*, 65–81.

Rink, E., Tricker, R., & Harvey, S. M. (2007). Onset of sexual intercourse among female adolescents: The influence of perceptions, depression, and ecological factors. *Journal of Adolescent Health, 41*(4), 398–406.

Roberts, D. F., Foehr, U. G., Rideout, V. J., & Brodie, M. (1999). Kids & media @ the New Millennium: A Kaiser Family Foundation Report: A Comprehensive National Analysis of Children's Media Use: Executive Summary. Menlo Park, CA: The Kaiser Family Foundation.

Rochon, J., Klesges, R. C., Story, M., Robinson, T. N., Baranowski, T., Obarzanek, E., et al. (2003) Common design elements of the Girls Health Enrichment Multi-site studies (GEMS). *Ethnicity and Disease, 13*(supplement), S6–14.

Romero, A. J. (2005). Low-income neighborhood barriers and resources for adolescents' physical activity. *Journal of Adolescent Health, 36*(3), 253–259.

Rose, A. J. & Montemayor, R. (1994). The relationship between gender role orientation and perceived self-competency in male and female adolescents. *Sex Roles, 31*(9–10), 579–595.

Rostosky, S. S., Danner, F., & Riggle, E. (2007). Is religiosity a protective factor against substance use in young adulthood? Only if you're straight! *Journal of Adolescent Health, 40*(5), 440–447

Rubenstein, A. & Zager, K. (2002). School, school, school – Why is there always a problem? In A. Rubenstein & K. Zager (Eds.), *The inside story on teen girls* (pp. 85–104). Washington, DC American Psychological Association.

Salazar, L. F., DiClemente, R. J., Wingood, G. M., Crosby, R. A., Harrington, K., Davis, S., et al. (2004). Self-concept and adolescents' refusal of unprotected sex: A test of mediating mechanisms among African American girls. *Prevention Science, 5(3)*, 137–149.

Santos, M., Richards, S. C., & Bleckley, K. M. (2007). Comorbidity between depression and disordered eating in adolescents. *Eating Behaviors, 8*(4), 440–449.

Scheffler, T. & Naus, P. (1999). The relationship between fatherly affirmation and a woman's self-esteem, fear of intimacy, comfort with womanhood, and comfort with sexuality. *The Canadian Journal of Human Sexuality, 8*, 39–45.

Schinke, S., Di Noia, J., Schwinn, T., & Cole, K. (2006). Drug abuse risk and protective factors among black urban adolescent girls: A group-randomized trial of computer-delivered mother-daughter intervention. *Psychology of Addictive Behaviors, 20*(4), 496–500.

Scott, K. A. (2004). African-American-White girls' friendships. *Feminism & Psychology, 14(3)*, 383–388.

See, L. A. & Larkin, R. (2007). The psychological effects of skin color on African Americans' self-esteem. In L. A. See (2nd ed.), *Human behavior in the social environment from an African American perspective* (pp. 153–181). New York, NY: Haworth Press.

Shields, A. & Cicchette, D. (2001). Parental maltreatment and emotional dysregulation as risk factors for bullying and victimization in middle childhood. *Journal of Clinical and Child Psychology, 30*(3), 349–363.

Siegel, J. M. (2002). Body image change and adolescent depressive symptoms. *Journal of Adolescent Research, 17*(1), 27–41.

Singh, K., Vaught, C., & Mitchell, C. W. (1999). Single-sex classes and academic achievement in two inner-city schools. *Journal of Negro Education, 67*(2), 157–167.

Sirin, S. R., & Rogers-Sirin, L. (2004). Exploring school engagement of middle-class African American adolescents. *Youth & Society, 35(3)*, 323–340.

Smalls, C., White, R., Chavous, T., & Sellers, R. (2007). Racial ideological beliefs and racial discriminations experiences as predictors of academic engagement among African American adolescents. *Journal of Black Psychology, 33(3)*, 299–330.

Smetana, J. G., Abernethy, A., & Harris, A. (2000). Adolescent-parent interations in middle class African American families: Longitudinal change and contextual variations. *Journal of Family Psychology, 14(3)*, 458–474.

Smetana, J. G. & Chuang, S. (2001). Middle-class African American parents' conceptions of parenting in early adolescence. *Journal of Research on Adolescence, 11(2)*, 177–198.

Smith, S. P. (1996). Dating-partner preferences among a group of inner-city African-American high school students. *Adolescence, 31*(121), 79–90.

Smith, J. R., Brooks-Gunn, J., & Klebanov, P. K. (2000). Welfare and work: Complementary strategies for low-income women. *Journal of Marriage and the Family, 62(3)*, 808–821.

Smith, C., Denton, M. L., Faris, R., & Regnerus, M. (2002). Spirituality and religiosity are considered aspects of prosocial behavior. *Journal for the Scientific Study of Religion,* (4), 597–612.

Smith, E. P., Walker, K., & Fields, L. (1999). Ethnic identity and its relationship to self-esteem, perceived efficacy and prosocial attitudes in early adolescence. *Journal of Adolescence, 22*(6), 867–880.

Solberg, M. E. & Olweus, D. (2003). Prevalence estimation of school bullying with the Oleweus Bully/Victim Questionnaire. *Aggressive Behavior, 29*, 239–268.

Sonya, N., Fung, M. T., & Trickett, M. T. (2008). Self-rated pubertal development, depressive symptoms and delinquency: Measurement issues and moderation by gender and maltreatment. *Journal of Youth and Adolescence, 37*(6), 736–746.

South, S. J. & Baumer, E. P. (2000). Deciphering community and race effects on adolescent premarital childbearing. *Social Forces, 78* (4), 1379–1408.

Spence, J. T., Helmreich, R. L., & Stapp, J. (1974). The Personal Attributes Questionnaire: A Measure of sex-role stereotypes and masculinity-femininity. *Journal Supplemental Abstract Service, Catalog of Selected Documents in Psychology, 4*, 43–44 (Ms. 617).

Steinberg, L. (1987). Single parents, stepparents, and the susceptibility of adolescents to antisocial peer pressure. *Child Development, 58*(1), 269–275.

Stephens, D. P. & Phillips, A. D. (2003). Freaks, gold diggers, divas, and dykes: The sociohistorical development of adolescent African American women's sexual script. *Sexuality and Culture: An Interdisciplinary Quarterly, 7*(1), 3–49.

Stevenson, H. (1995). Relationship of adolescent perceptions of racial socialization to racial identity. *Journal of Black Psychology, 21*(1), 49–70.

St. Lawrence, J. S., Brasfield, T. L., Jefferson, K. W., et al. (1995). Cognitive-behavioral intervention to reduce African American adolescent risk for HIV infection. *Journal of Consulting and Clinical Psychology, 63*, 221–237.

Stolberg, M. E. & Olweus, D. (2003). Prevalence estimation of school bullying with the Oleweus Bully/Victim Questionnaire. *Aggressive Behavior, 29*, 239–268.

Stolley, M. R. & Fitzgibbon, M. L. (1997). Effects of an obesity prevention program on the eating behavior of African American mothers and daughters. *Health Education & Behavior, 24*, 152–164.

Strasburger, V. C. (1997). 'Sex, drugs, rock 'n' roll' and the media: Are the media responsible for adolescent behavior? *Adolescent Medicine, 8*, 403–414.

Striegel-Moore, R. H., Dohm, F., Kraemer, H.C., Taylor, C., Daniels, S., Crawford, P. B., et al., (2003). Eating disorders in white and black women. *The American Journal of Psychiatry, 160*, 1326–1331.

Striegel-Moore, R. H., Wilfley, D.E., Pike. K. M, Dohm, F., & Fairburn, C. G. (2000). *Archives of Family Medicine, 9*, 83–87.

Substance Abuse and Mental Health Services Administration (2002). *2002 National Survey on Drug Use and Health*. Rockville, MA: US.

Substance Abuse and Mental Health Services Administration (SAMHSA). (2005). *Results from the 2004 national survey on drug use and health: National findings* (Office of Applied Studies, NSDUH). Rockville, MD.

Surgeon General's Report on Mental Health (1999), U.S. Health and Human Services. Retrieved on October 10, 2008 from http://mentalhealth.samhsa.gov/cmhs/surgeongeneral/surgeongeneralrpt.asp

Taylor, R., Chatters, L., & Levin, J. (2004). *Religion in the lives of African-Americans: Social, psychological and health perspectives*. Thousand Oaks: Sage Publications.

Taylor-Seehafer, M. & Rew, L. (2000). Risky sexual behavior among adolescent women. *Journal of the Society of Pediatric Nurses, 5*(1), 15–25.

Tesser, A. (1988). Toward a self-evaluation maintenance model of social behavior. *Advances in Experimental Social Psychology, 21*, 181–227.

Thoman, E. (1998). *Skills and strategies for media education*. Los Angeles, CA: Center for Media Literacy.

Thomas, D.E. & Bierman, K. L. (2006). The impact of classroom aggression on the development of aggressive behavior problems in children. *Development and Psychopathology, 18*, 471–487.

Thomas, A.J. & King, C. T. (2007). Gendered racial socialization of African American mothers and daughters. *The Family Journal, 15*(2), 137–142.

Thornton, M. C. (1997). Strategies of racial socialization among Black parents: Mainstream, minority, and cultural messages. In R.J. Taylor, J.S. Jackson, & L.M. Chatters (Eds.), *Family Life in Black America* (pp. 201–215). Thousand Oaks, CA: Sage.

Tolson, J. M. & Urberg, K. A. (1993). Similarity between adolescent best friends. *Journal of Adolescent Research, 8*(3), 274–288.

Townsend, T.G. & Belgrave, F.Z. (2000). The impact of personal identity and racial identity on drug attitudes and use among African American children. *Journal of Black Psychology, 26*(4), 421–436.

Travis, C.B. & White, J.W. (2000). Sexual roles of girls and women: An ethnocultural lifespan perspective. In Reid & Bing (Eds.), *Sexuality, Society, and Feminism* (pp. 141–161). Washington, DC: APA.

Turiel, E. & Neff, K. (2000). Religion, culture, and beliefs about reality in moral reasoning. In
  K. S. Rosengen, C. N. Johnson, & P. L. Harris (Eds.). *Imagining the impossible: Magical, scien-
  tific, and religious thinking in children* (pp. 269–304). Cambridge, UK: Cambridge University
  Press.
Unger, J. B., Rohrbach, L. A., Cruz, T. B., Baexconde-Garbanati, L., Howard, K. A., Palmer, P. H.
  et al.(2001). Ethnic variation in peer influences on adolescent smoking. *Nicotine & Tobacco
  Research, 3(2)*, 167–176.
Upchurch, D. M., Aneshensel, C. S., Sucoff, C. A., & Levy-Storms, L. (1999). Neighborhood and
  family contexts of adolescent sexual activity. *Journal of Marriage & the Family, 61(4)*,
  920–933.
U.S. Bureau of Labor Statistics (2009). *Employment Status of the Civilion Populationby Race, Sex,
  and Age.* Retrieved May 29, 2009, from http://www.bls.gov/news.release/empsit.t02.htm
U.S. Bureau of Labor Statistics Division of Current Employment. Retrieved October 13, 2008,
  from www.bls.gov/news.release/empsit.t02.htm
US Census Bureau (2000). *Census 2000 Urban and Rural Classification.* Retrieved October 10,
  2008 from http://www.census.gov/geo/www/ua/ua_2k.html
U.S. Census Bureau (2006). American Community Survey. Retrieved July 21, 2008, from
  http://factfinder.census.gov/servlet/DatasetMainPageServlet?_program=ACS&_submenuId=
  datasets_2&_lang=en&_ts=
US Census Bureau (2007). American Community Survey: The American Community-Blacks:
  2004. Retrieved May 29, 2009 from http://www.census.gov/prod/2007pubs/acs-04.pdf
US Census Bureau (2007). *National Population Estimates-Characteristics. Table 3: Annual Esti-
  mates of the Population by Sex, Race, and Hispanic or Latino Origin for the United States:
  April 1, 200 to July 1, 2006.* Retrieved May 17, 2007, from http://www.census.gov/popest/
  national/asrh/NC-EST2006-srh.html
U.S. Census Bureau (2004, March 14). *Presence of grandparents in house by race.* Retrieved
  July 21, 2008, from http://factfinder.census.gov.
U.S. Census Bureau (2007) Table 3: Annual Estimates of the Population by Sex, Race and Hispanic
  or Latino Origin for the United States: April 1, 2000 to July 1, 2006. Retrieved May 17, 2007
  from http://www.census.gov/popest/national/asrh/NCEST2006/
U.S. Census Bureau (2004) Community Survey, Selected Population profiles, S0201.
U.S. Department of Commerce, Census Bureau, Current Population Survey (CPS), October
  (1972–2005).
U.S. Department of Commerce, Census Bureau. (2005). *Status dropout rates of 16- through
  24-year-olds, by sex and race/ethnicity.* Current Population Survey (CPS), October (1972–
  2005).
U.S. Department of Education, National Center for Education Statistics. (2005). *Gender
  differences in participation and completion of undergraduate education and how they have
  changed over time* (NCES 2005-169). Washington, DC: U.S. Government Printing Office:
  K. Peter, L. Horn.
U.S. Department of Education, National Center for Education Statistics. (2001). *Dropout rates in
  the United States: 2000* (NCES 2002114). Washington, DC: U.S. Government Printing Office.
U.S. Health and Human Services. Surgeon General's Report on Mental Health (1999), Reprieved
  from Parke, R., & Buriel, R. (1998). Socialization in the family: Ethnic and ecological perspectives. In W. Damon & N. Eisenberg (Eds.), *Handbook of Child Psychology: Social, Emotional
  and personality development. 5th ed.. Vol. 3.* (pp. 463–552). Hoboken, NJ: John Wiley & Sons,
  Inc.
Ventura, S. J., Abma, J. C., Mosher, W. D., & Henshaw, S. K. (2006). *Recent trends in teenage
  pregnancy in the United States, 1990–2002.* Health E-stats. Hyattsville, MD: National Center
  for Health Statistics.
Wallace, J. M. (1998). Explaining race differences in adolescent and young adult drug use: The
  role of racialized social systems. *Drugs & Society, 14(1)*, 21–36.

Wallace, J. M., Bachman, J. G., O'Malley, P. M., Schulenberg, J. E., Cooper, S. M., & Johnston, L. D. (2003). Gender and ethnic differences in smoking, drinking, and illicit drug use among American 8th, 10th, and 12th grade students, 1976–2000. *Addiction, 98*(2), 225–234.

Wallace, J. M. & Muroff, J. R. (2002). Preventing substance abuse among African American children and youth: Race differences in risk factor exposure and vulnerability. *The Journal of Primary Prevention, 22*(3), 235–261.

Walker-Barnes, C. J. & Mason, C. A. (2001). Perceptions of risk factors for female gang involvement among African American and Hispanic women. *Youth & Society, 32*(3), 303–336.

Wang, H., Kao, G., & Joyner, K. (2006). Stability of interracial and intraracial romantic relationships among adolescents. *Social Science Research, 35(2)*, 435–453.

Ward, L. M. (2004). Wading through the stereotypes: Positive and negative associations between media use and Black adolescents' conception of self. *Developmental Psychology, 40*(2), 284–294.

Way, N. (1995). "Can't you see the courage, the strength that I have?": Listening to urban adolescent girls speak about their relationships. *Psychology of Women Quarterly, 19*, 107–128.

Way, N. (1996). Between experiences of betrayal and desire: Close friendships among urban adolescents. In B. J. Ross & N. Way (Eds.), *Urban girls: Resisting stereotypes, creating identities*. New York: University Press.

Way, N. & Gillman, D. (2000). Early adolescent girls' perceptions of their relationship with their fathers: A qualitative investigation. *Journal of Early Adolescence, 20*, 309–331.

Wentzel, K. R., Filisetti, L., & Looney, L. (2007). Adolescent prosocial behavior: The role of self-processes and contextual cues. *Child Development, 78*(3), 895–910.

White, K. S., Bruce, S. E., Farrell, A. D., & Kliewer, W. (1998). Impact of exposure to community violence on anxiety: A longitudinal study of family social support as a protective factor for urban children. *Journal of Child and Family Studies, 7*(2), 187–203.

Wingood, G. M., Diclemente, R. J., & Harrington, K. (2002). Body image of African American females' sexual health. *Journal of Women's Health and Gender-based Medicine, 11*(5), 433–439.

Womenshealth.gov (2008). *Eating disorders information fact sheet: African American girls*. Retrieved July 31, 2008, from www.womenshealth.gov/bodyimage/kids/bodywise/uf/African-AmericanGirls.pdf

Wood, D., Kaplan, R., & McLoyd, V. C. (2007). Gender differences in the educational expectations of urban, low-income African American youth: The role of parents and the school. *Journal of Youth Adolescence, 36*, 417–427.

Woods, L. N. & Jagers, R. J. (2003). Are cultural values predictors of moral reasoning in African American adolescents? *Journal of Black Psychology, 29*(1), 102–118.

Woodhill, B. M. & Samuels, C. A. (2003). Positive and negative androgyny and their relationship with psychological health and well-being. *Sex Roles, 48*(11–12), 555–565.

Wong, C. A., Eccles, J. S., & Sameroff, A. (2003). The influence of ethnic discrimination and ethnic identification on African American adolescents' school and socioemotional adjustment. *Journal of Personality, 71*(6), 1197–1232.

Wu, A. C., Smith, L., Bokhour, B., Hohman, K. H., & Lieu, T. A. (2008). Racial/ethnic variation in parent perceptions of asthma. *Ambulatory Pediatrics, 8*(2), 89–97.

Young-Hyman, D., Schlundt, D. G., Herman, L., De Luca, F., & Counts, D. (2001). Evaluations of the insulin resistance syndrome in 5- to 10- year old overweight/obese African-American children. *Diabetes Care, 24*, 1359–1364.

Zimmer-Gembeck, M. J., Siebenbruner, J., & Collins, W. A. (2001). Diverse aspects of dating: Associations with psychosocial functioning from early to middle adolescence. *Journal of Adolescence, 24*, 313–336.

Index

CPSIA information can be obtained at www.ICGtesting.com
Printed in the USA
LVOW10s1719060916

503446LV00009B/80/P